Bisphenols

Edited by Pınar Erkekoğlu

Published in London, United Kingdom

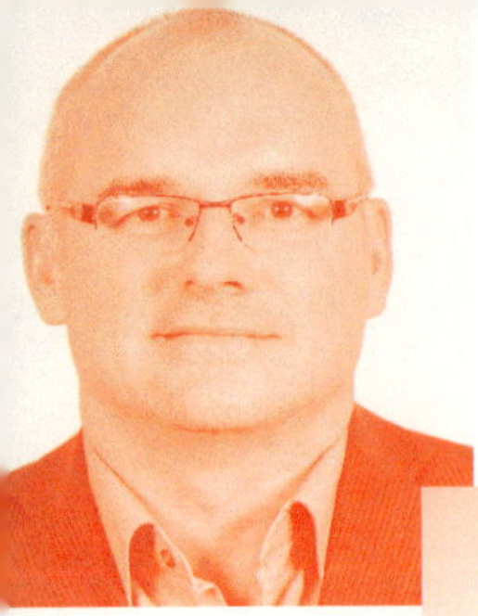
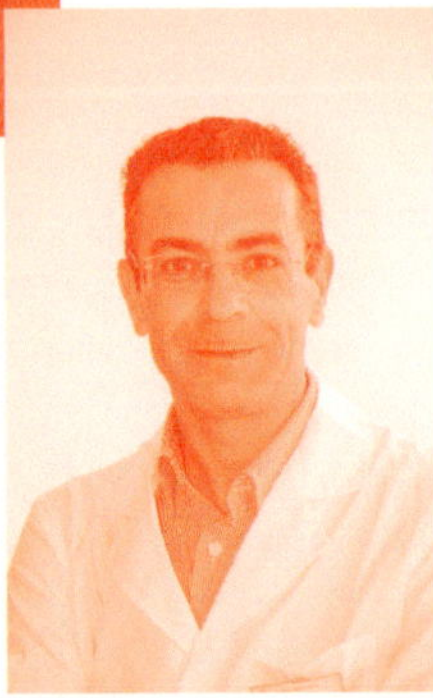
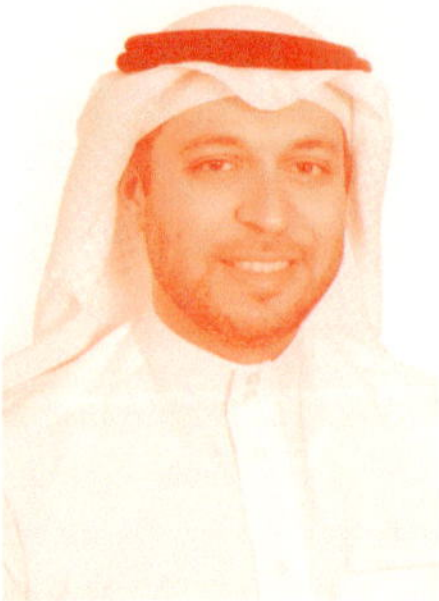
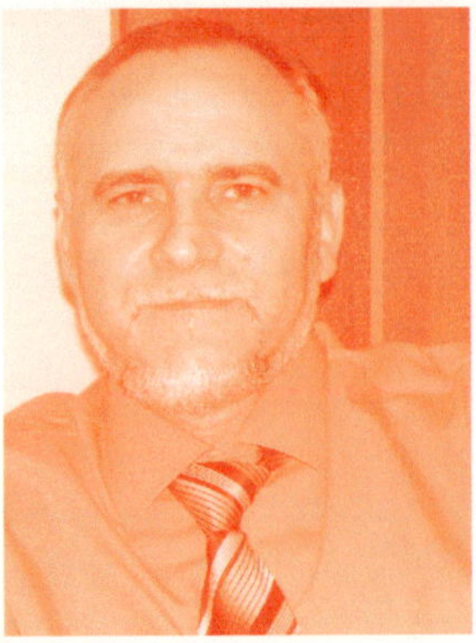
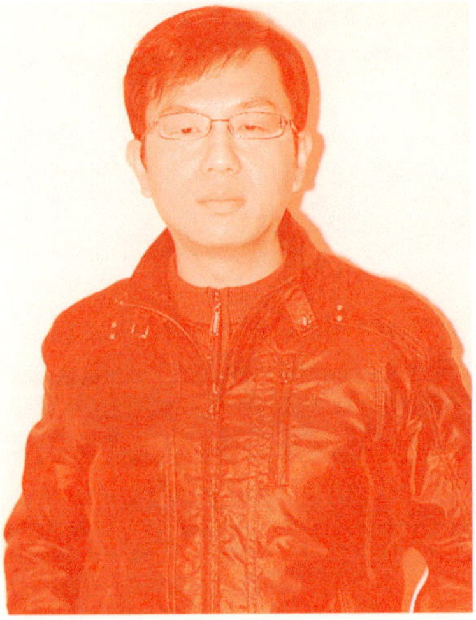
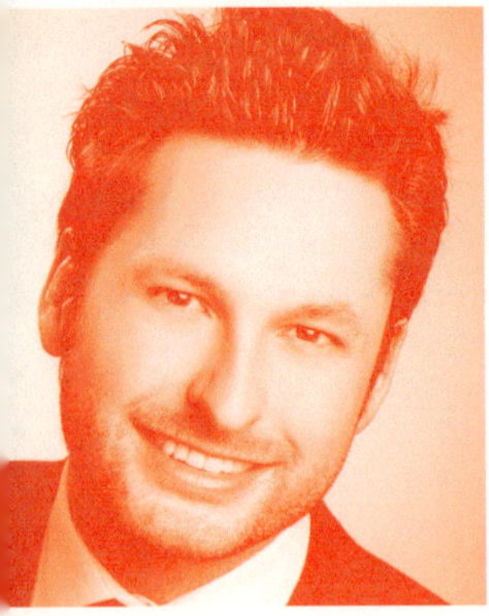
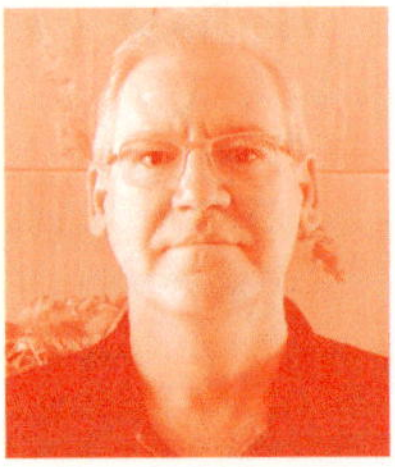

IntechOpen

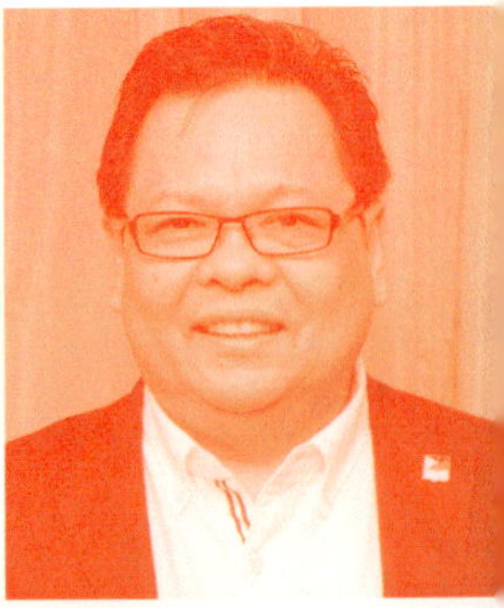
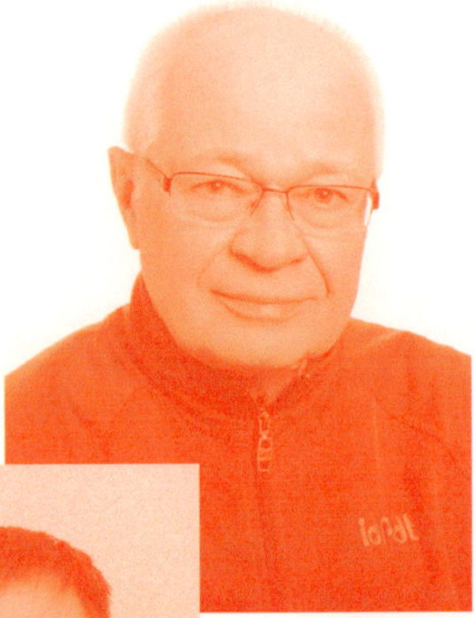
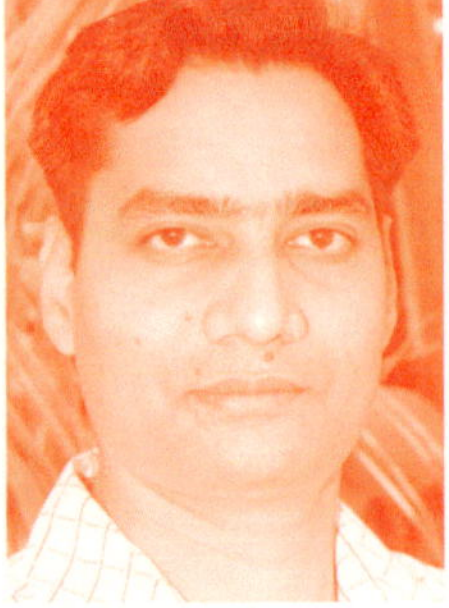
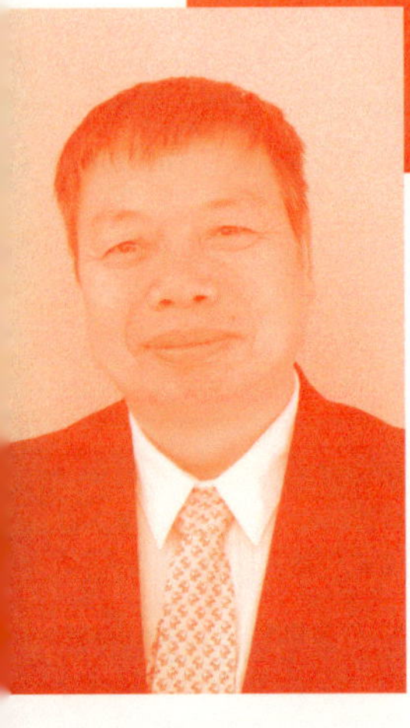
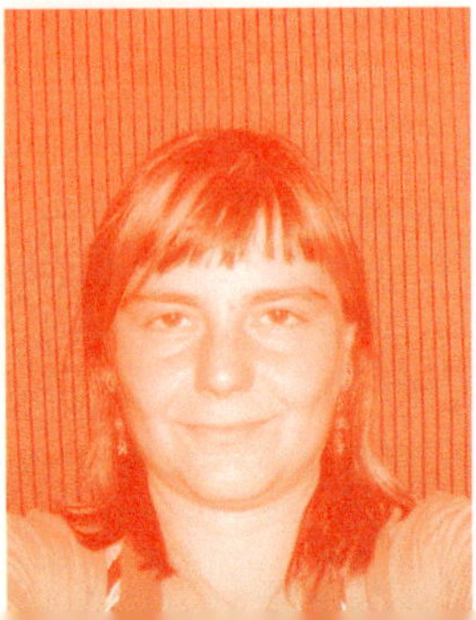
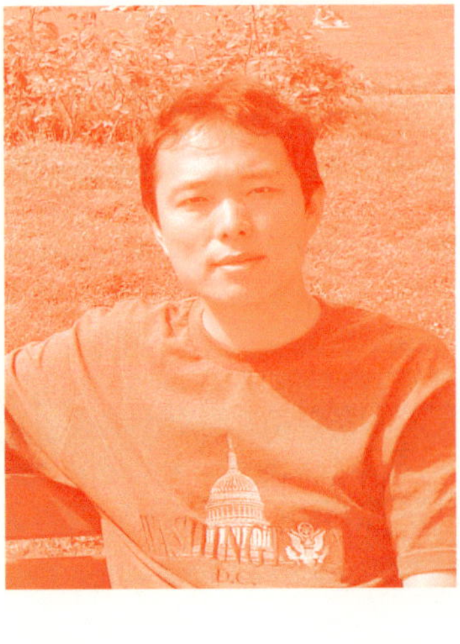

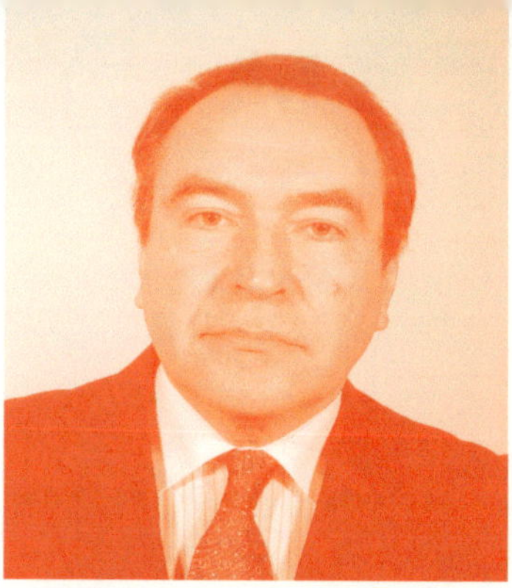

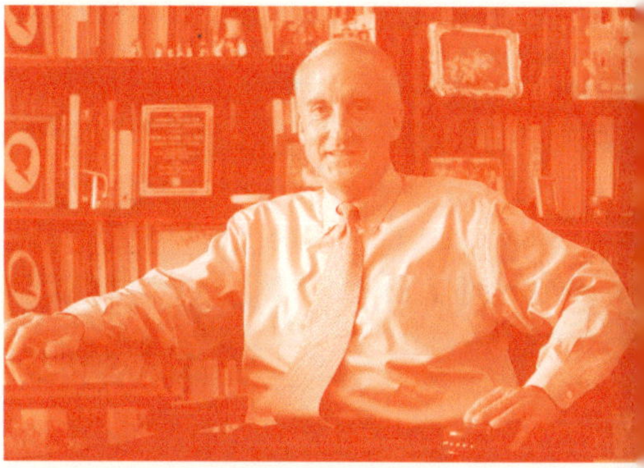

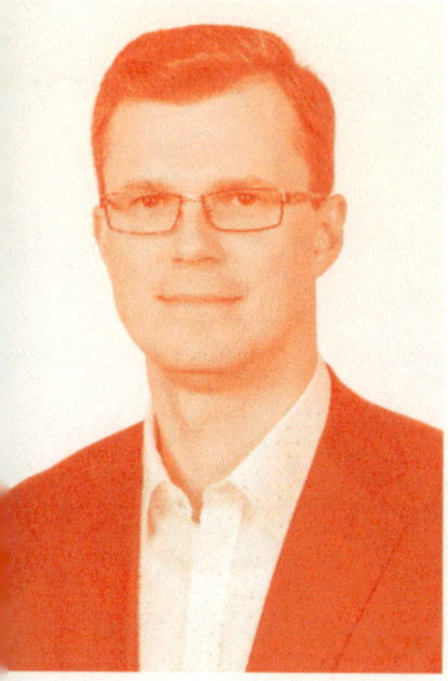

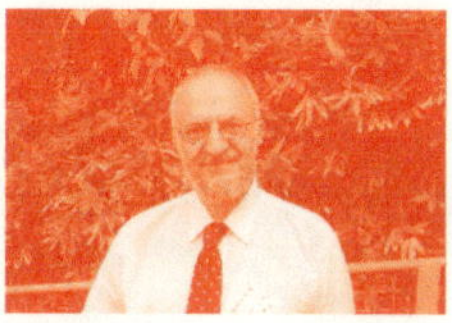

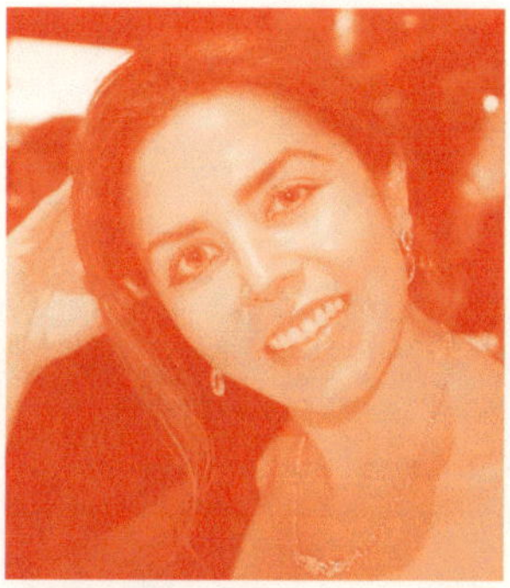

Supporting open minds since 2005

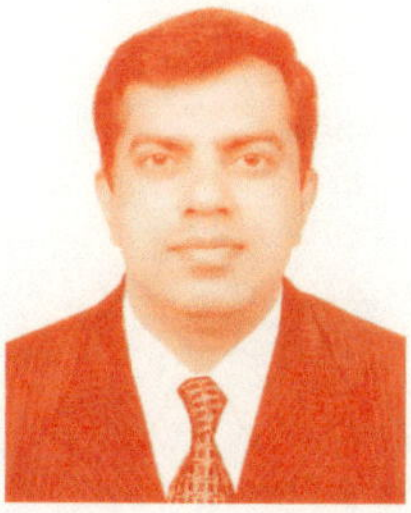

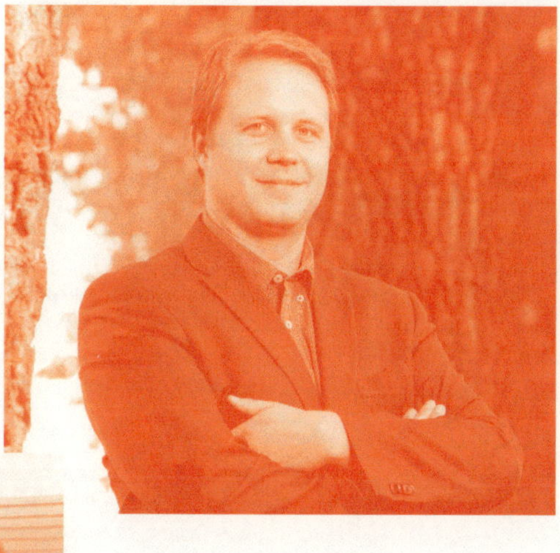

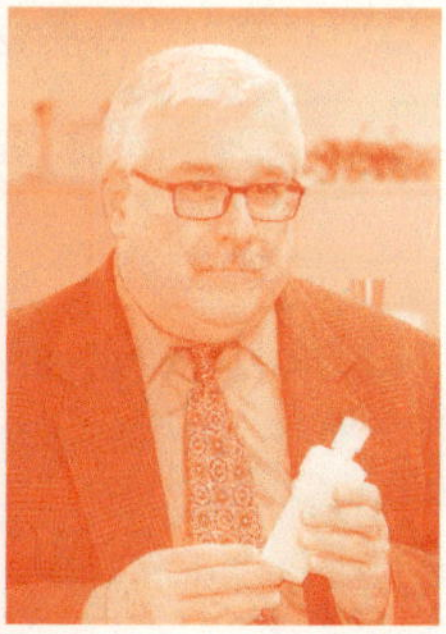

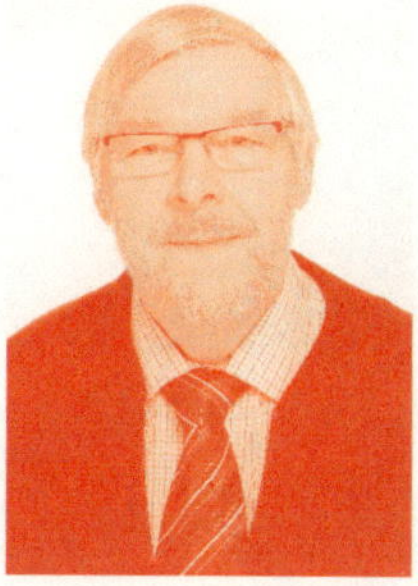

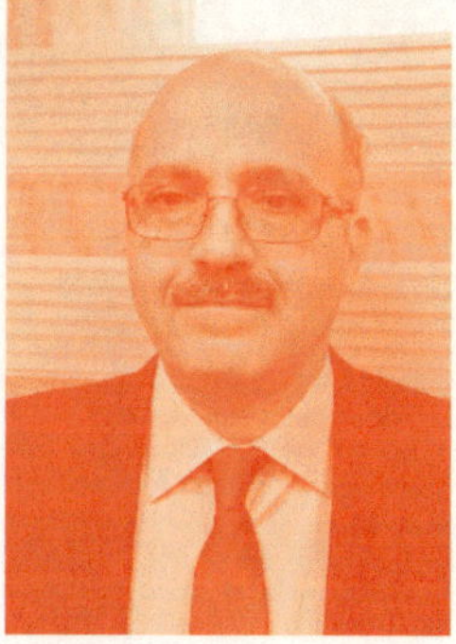

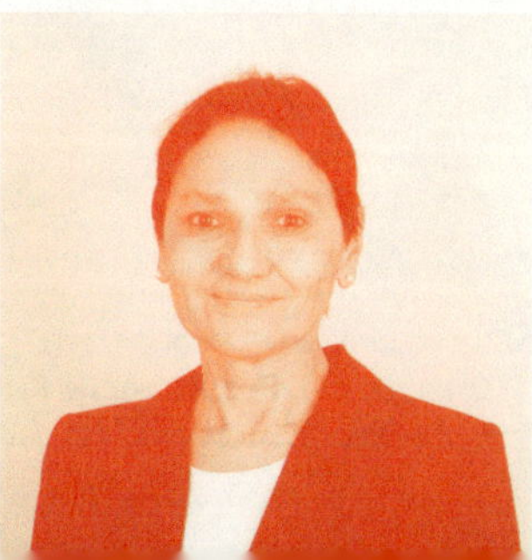

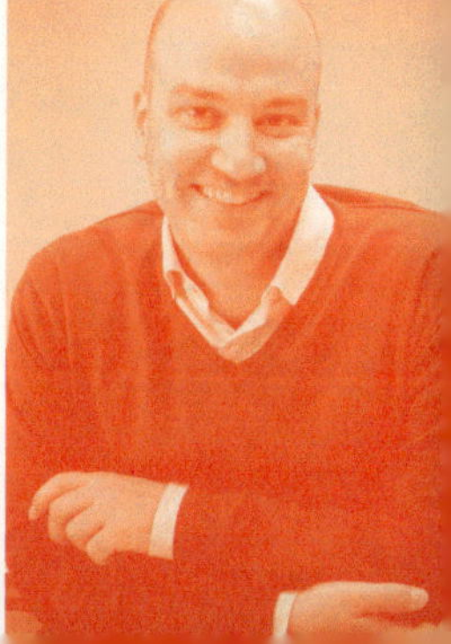

Bisphenols
http://dx.doi.org/10.5772/intechopen.95193
Edited by Pınar Erkekoğlu

Contributors
Geethamani Palanisamy, Divya Palanisamy, Zouhour Hsine, Rym Mlika, Ali Olfati, Parichehr Nouri, Budiawan, Intan Cahaya Dani, Sri Handayani, Chrissy Fransisca Olivyana Rugian, Luis Molina, Pamela Ehrenfeld, Carlos D. Figueroa, Pınar Erkekoğlu, Anıl Yirün, Aylin Balcı Özyurt

First published in London, United Kingdom, 2022 by IntechOpen
IntechOpen is the global imprint of INTECHOPEN LIMITED, registered in England and Wales, registration number: 11086078, 5 Princes Gate Court, London, SW7 2QJ, United Kingdom
Printed in Croatia

British Library Cataloguing-in-Publication Data
A catalogue record for this book is available from the British Library

Additional hard and PDF copies can be obtained from orders@intechopen.com

Bisphenols
Edited by Pınar Erkekoğlu
p. cm.
Print ISBN 978-1-83969-541-4
Online ISBN 978-1-83969-542-1
eBook (PDF) ISBN 978-1-83969-543-8

For EU product safety concerns:
IN TECH d.o.o., Prolaz Marije Krucifikse Kozulić 3, 51000 Rijeka, Croatia, info@intechopen.com or visit our website at intechopen.com.

Meet the editor

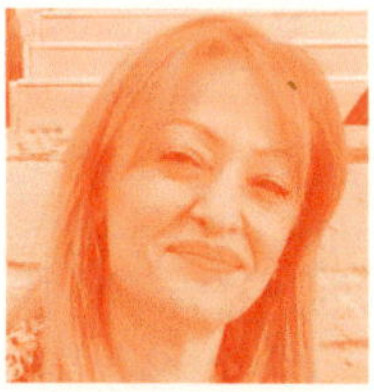

Pınar Erkekoğlu graduated from the Faculty of Pharmacy, Hacettepe University, Turkey, where she received her MSci and Ph.D. in Toxicology. She completed her Ph.D. studies at the University of Joseph Fourier, France, and the French Alternative Energies and Atomic Energy Commission/Institute for Nanosciences and Cryogenics/Nucleic Acid Lesions (CEA/INAC/LAN). She worked as a post-doc and visiting associate in the Biological Engineering Department, Massachusetts Institute of Technology (MIT), USA. She is currently a full professor and head of the Department of Toxicology, Hacettepe University, and a faculty staff/board member at the Hacettepe University Vaccine Institute. Her main interests are endocrine-disrupting chemicals, neurotoxic chemicals, and the toxic effects of vaccines. Dr. Erkekoğlu has published more than 180 papers and 15 book chapters. She has edited seven international books and served as the translation editor for three others. She has been a European Registered Toxicologist (ERT) since 2014.

Contents

Preface

Bisphenols are a group of chemicals that have been used to manufacture plastics, epoxy resins, and other products since the 1960s. Humans are exposed to these chemicals via ingestion, inhalation, or medical procedures.

Bisphenol-A (BPA) was initially investigated for pharmaceutical use as a synthetic estrogen in the 1930s and today it is suggested to be a weakly estrogenic "endocrine disruptor." The results of some recent studies, in which animals were exposed to low doses of this chemical, describe subtle effects in laboratory animals.

BPA was found to be present in urine, amniotic fluid, and breast milk according to the results of several well-conducted studies in humans. BPA may cause reproductive, developmental, and systemic toxic effects and there are questions about its potential impact, particularly on children's health and the environment. Due to these concerns, the Food and Drug Administration (FDA) and the Canadian government have banned BPA in baby formula packaging, infant bottles, and sippy cups, but declared it safe for other uses. France has the strictest BPA regulations in Europe and the French government has banned BPA in all food and beverage packaging and utensils since 2015. The European Union expanded its restrictions on the use of BPA in food packaging, building on a previous ban of the chemical in infant bottles. BPA containing thermal receipts ($\geq 0.02\%$) is no longer sold in Europe, effectively banning its use. The Environmental Protection Agency (EPA) says it has no plans to introduce BPA regulations, though it has raised concerns over its health and environmental effects.

There are several alternatives to BPA today, although they also have a "bisphenol" structure. For example, bisphenol S (BPS) and bisphenol F (BPF) are widely used in products that are labeled as "BPA-free." BPS is generally more tolerant to heat and is more photo-resistant than BPA. BPS is used in fast-drying epoxy glues, as a corrosion inhibitor, and a reactant in polymer reactions. BPS is also present in thermal receipts, mailing envelopes, tickets, airplane boarding passes, and luggage tags.

BPF, on the other hand, is used in the production of plastics, lacquers, structural adhesives, the inner lining of soda cans, dental materials, grouts, coatings, tank/pipe linings, industrial flooring, road and bridge deck toppings, and electrical varnishes. BPF is also utilized in liners, adhesives, plastics, and the coating of drinks and food cans. Although there are not yet as many studies on these alternatives as there are on BPA, the results of different in vitro and in vivo research suggest that these alternatives may also lead to toxic effects. Therefore, both BPS and BPF cannot be considered "safe," and more research should be conducted in order to understand their mechanisms of toxicity in different organs and systems. Moreover, their use should be restricted like that of BPA if they are suggested to cause toxicity in susceptible populations, particularly in babies and young children.

This book focuses on the pathological conditions that may be caused by bisphenol derivatives, detection methods, and regulations in different countries. It presents information on the mechanisms of toxicity of bisphenols and the suggestions of regulatory authorities for the use of bisphenol derivatives in different user products. This book is a valuable reference for readers who want detailed knowledge on the reproductive toxicity of BPA and its alternatives.

Dr. Pınar Erkekoğlu
Professor,
Faculty of Pharmacy,
Department of Toxicology,
Hacettepe University,
Ankara, Turkey

Section 1

Molecular Effects of Bisphenols

Chapter 1

In Vivo Study of DNA Adduct (8-OHdG) Formation of *Rattus novergicus* Using Bisphenol a through Fenton-Like Reaction and Nickel (II) as Cancer Risk Biomarker

Budiawan, Intan Cahaya Dani,
Chrissy Fransisca Olivyana Rugian and Sri Handayani

Abstract

Bisphenol A (BPA) has been used in many consumer products including plastics, and food packaging. There is the evidence that Bisphenol A have potential to cause oxidative stress by disturbing the redox status in cells. We have conducted the in vivo study of BPA and Ni(II) exposure to *Rattus novergicus* and confirmed the formation of DNA adduct 8-OHdG as biomarker of oxidative stress and cancer risk. Subacute dose of BPA (2 mg/kg BW) and Ni (II) metals (0.1 μg/kg BW) have been exposed to animal test for 28 days. We collected the urine sample of animal samples every week. The formation of 8-OHdG found in urine of animal samples monitored by Liquid Chromatography–Mass Spectrometry (LC–MS/MS). The result of this study indicates that levels of 8-OHdG in animal samples exposed to BPA and BPA-Ni (II) increase every week. However, levels of 8-OHdG in animal samples exposed by BPA-Ni (II) is less than levels of 8-OHdG in animal samples exposed by BPA only. This can be happened because Ni (II) given to animal samples are not in the excessed levels, therefore the synergic effect of BPA and Ni (II) has not already been seen. The hydroxyl radical can cause oxidative DNA damage and interact with DNA guanine base by producing DNA adduct 8-hydroxy-2′-deoxyguanosine (8-OHdG). This book aimed to obtain information regarding in vivo study of BPA and metal ions exposure can generate hydroxyl radical as a dominant form of Reactive Oxygen Species (ROS) that can interact with macromolecules such as DNA and form DNA adduct as biomarker of oxidative stress and cancer risk.

Keywords: BPA, Nickel (II), 8-OHdG, in vivo study

1. Introduction

Bisphenol A (BPA) is a common chemical compound with the highest production volume in worldwide [1]. BPA is a synthetic chemical used as a monomer for the manufacture of polycarbonate plastic, and also as an intermediate in the synthesis of epoxy resins. Humans have considerable possibilities for direct exposure to BPA from plastic beverage containers and from saliva patients receiving dental fillings [2]. Humans are exposed to BPA through their diet, inhalation of household dust, and dermal exposure [3]. Bisphenol A (BPA) is a known endocrine disruptor [4]. It have a potent reproductive and genotoxic agent and affects the normal physiological functions [5]. Oxidative stress has been proven as a basic mechanism of BPA toxicity in animal models for years. Bisphenol A have the potential to cause oxidative stress by disturbing the redox status in cells [6].

On the other side, heavy metals Nickel (II), may contribute to the formation of ROS in humans. Humans may be exposed to nickel if involved in nickel production or through contact with everyday items such as nickel-containing jewelry, tableware, and cigarettes. Ni (II) is toxic and carcinogenic in animals and humans [7] and has been classified by the International Agency for Research on Cancer (IARC) as a carcinogen in humans [8]. This can be happened because nickel ions (II) also have the ability to form hydroxyl radicals through Fenton-like reactions [9].

The hydroxyl radicals formed can cause oxidative stress. Such increased oxidative stress can lead to DNA damage which can result in carcinogenesis [10–13]. In DNA repair, additional products are formed and released into the bloodstream and appears in the urine without further metabolism. The 8-hydroxy-2'deoxiguanosine (8-OHdG) compound is one of the adducts derived from the hydroxyl radical attack

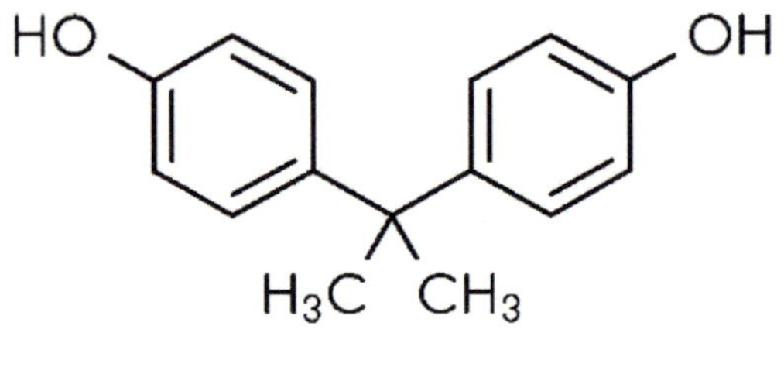

Figure 1.
Structure of bisphenol A.

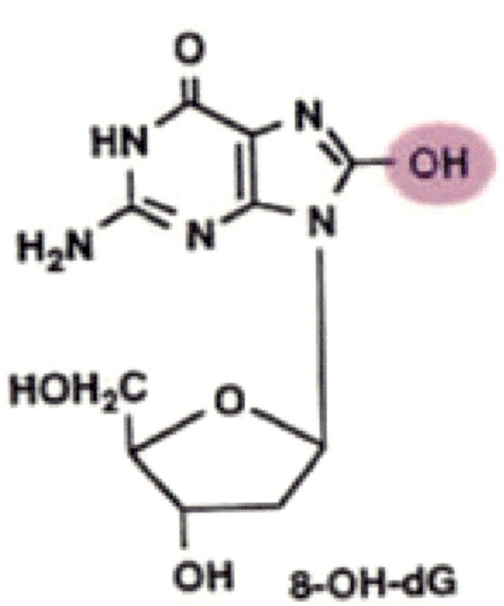

Figure 2.
Structure of 8-OHdG.

of deoxyguanosine residue and has been commonly used as a biomarker of oxidative damage to DNA [14]. With the detection of 8-OHdG, the risk of cancer can be detected earlier so that it can be further minimized.

This study aims to determine the formation of 8-OHdG which is an indicator of DNA damage due to exposure from BPA and Nickel (II) metal (**Figures 1** and **2**). The 8-OHdG in vivo formation was analyzed in the urine of Sprague–Dawley rats. For analysis of 8-OHdG, pre-treatment method of urine sample with SPE (Solid Phase Extraction) was performed. Furthermore, an analysis using LC–MS/MS instrument is used to view and analyze the formation of 8-OHdG as a proof of exposure of those toxic substances which can lead to DNA damage.

2. Experimental methods

2.1 Materials

The materials used for the rats' exposure rats are Bisphenol A (BPA), Nickel (II) metal in the form of $NiCl_2.6H_2O$. 8-hydroxy-2′-deoxyguanosine, ammonium acetate, acetic acid, acetonitrile, aquabidest, methanol, and SPE cartridge SPE *SUPELCO-Discovery® DSC*-18.

2.2 In vivo study

2.2.1 Experimental animals

In this study, the experimental animals used were 8-weeks old male white rats from the Sprague–Dawley strain, weighed approximately between 120 and 220 grams obtained from the Faculty of Animal Husbandry of Non Ruminants and Animal Hope, Bogor Agricultural Institute, Bogor. Prior to the research, rats were acclimatized for 7 days so that they could adapt to the new environment. Then, all of the rats were adjusted to the optimal weight for 14 days. The food were pellets and placed in a cage while drinking water were given at the drinking place by pipette - *ad libitum*.

2.2.2 Xenobiotics exposure to experimental animals

Rats as experimental animals were divided into several groups. The groups were: Group A (group of rats with no exposure or control), group B (group of rats exposed to BPA), and group C (group of rats exposed to BPA and Ni (II). Each group consists of 5 rats. The study was conducted for 28 days. All the exposures were done by oral route (syringes equipped with a blunt-shaped or blunt-shaped cannula). The dose for each group of experimental animals are given in **Table 1**.

2.2.3 Urine sampling

The urine samples were used for the 8-OHdG analysis. For urine collection, rats were placed in a metabolic cage. When the urine is fully contained in the container located in the metabolism cage, urine is transferred to the micro-tube and then stored at −20°C freezer until the time for measurement using LC–MS/MS.

2.3 LC–MS/MS

Samples were analyzed on a 20A high performance liquid chromatography system (Shimadzu, Japan) coupled with an AB Sciex Q-Trap 3200 mass

Dose in each group	BPA	Ni (II)
Group A	—	—
Group B	2 mg/kg bw	—
Group C	2 mg/kg bw	0,1 μg/kg bw
bw: body weight.		

Table 1.
Dose of xenobiotics exposed to experimental animals.

Time (minutes)	Pump B Concentration (%)
0	0
0.5	5
1	95
2	95
2.5	5
3	0

Table 2.
Eluent gradient on LC–MS/MS.

Parameter	Precursor Ion	Q3 (Product Ion)	
	284,1	168,2	140,1
Q1	DP	43	43
	EP	4	4
MRM	CE	17	40
	CXP	3	3

Table 3.
Optimization result for LC–MS/MS instrument to measure 8-OHdG.

spectrometer and were separated on a Hypersil Gold C18 column (50 x 2,1 mm, 5 μm, Thermo Scientific). The pump used is in gradient mode. The mobile phase composition (eluent) is Ammonium Acetate 20 mM pH 4 (Pump A) and Acetonitrile (Pump B) which were adjusted automatically during elution with a gradient of 5–95% Acetonitrile solution with a certain time setting. **Table 2** shows the mobile phase (eluent) gradient during elution:

The flow rate used is 0.5 mL/min. Meanwhile, the column temperature is set at 40°C. The sample injected was as much as 10 μL and the analysis time was 5 minutes. The MS/MS parameters, including parent ion (Q1), product ion (Q3), collision energies (CE), declustering potential (DP), entrance potential (EP) and collision exit potential (CXP) were optimized. The optimized parameters are listed in **Table 3**.

Determination of 8-OHdG calibration curve was done by making standard series of each 10 μL 8-OHdG standard solution at concentration of 1 ng / mL (ppb), 5 ng / mL, 10 ng / mL, 25 ng / mL, 50 ng/mL. Measurements were made for each of these standard concentrations to obtain a calibration curve between the peak area obtained from the standard solution concentration, with a straight-line equation having

$R^2 > 0.996$. Limit of Detection (LOD) and Limit of Quantification (LOQ) limits are performed statistically by linear regression of the calibration curve. The measurement value will be equal to the value of b on the linear line y = a + bx, whereas the standard deviation of the blank is equal to the residual standard deviation (S (y/x)).

2.4 Analysis of 8-OHdG in urine samples

500 μL of urine samples were passed to the SPE SUPELCO -Discovery® DSC-18 cartridge column, previously conditioned with 5 ml of methanol and 5 ml of Ammonium Acetate. Furthermore, the cartridge was rinsed with 20 mM Ammonium Acetate pH 4: Acetonitrile (97: 3) of 5 ml. Samples are streamed to the SPE column of 500 μL. The fraction containing 8-OHdG in the cartridge is dried with N2 gas under vacuum SUPELCO VISIPREP. The fraction was added Ammonium Acetate 20 mM pH 4: Acetonitrile (80:20) of 5 ml. The elution results are then dried with nitrogen gas. A total of 10 μL samples were injected into the LC–MS/MS instrument to analyze its 8-OHdG formation.

3. Results and discussion

3.1 Determination of optimal conditions for 8-OHdG formation using LC–MS

Prior to the analysis of 8-OHdG formation in urine samples, optimization was done in advance to determine the best condition of the instrument, resulting in a performance of the method with good sensitivity. For the mobile phase, 20 mM Ammonium acetate with pH 4 and acetonitrile was used according to the method in the literature [15]. In **Figure 3**, from the standard 8-OHdG 50 ppb measurement results, it can be seen that 8-OHdG appears at retention time of 0.738 minutes.

3.1.1 Optimization of mass spectrometer condition

In LC–MS/MS instrument it takes at least two ion products with the highest intensity. This is useful for quantitative information in which the molecular weight compound is detected by the instrument in peak form, and to provide confirmation that the resulting peak actually belongs to the desired compound.

Figure 4(a) shows that the 8-OHdG compound is detected by Q1 to produce a precursor ion value of 284. Then, the ions are split in the presence of accelerated ions by the gas which in this LC–MS/MS instrument is nitrogen gas. Therefore, the

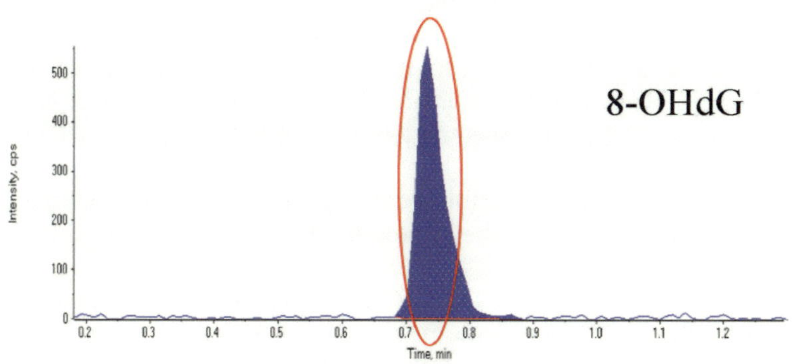

Figure 3.
Chromatogram of 8-OHdG standard (50 ppb).

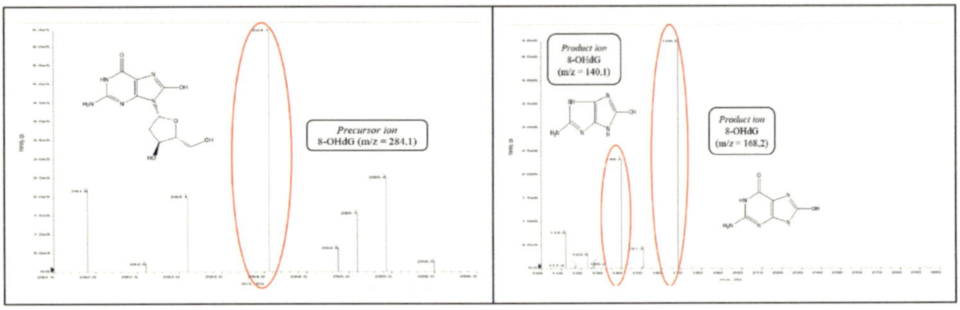

Figure 4.
(a) *The ion precursor of the 8-OHdG compound with Q1 detection (m/z = 284.1)* **(b)** *the product ion of 8-OHdG (m/z = 168.2) and (m/z = 140.1).*

precursor ions will be broken down into smaller ion fragments of molecular weight, which are further fragmented in Q3 to produce the highest intensity productions at 168.2. The transition for the selected mass spectrometer for 8-OHdG is m/z 284.1 → 168.2 for quantification and m/z 284.1 → 140.1 for qualification. Product ion 168,2 and 140,1 can be seen in **Figure 4(b)**.

8-OHdG with m/z 284,1 is fragmented into its product ions 168,2 and 140,1 according to **Figure 4(b)**. First, there is a cutting of sugar in the 8-OHdG compound, which causes 8-OHdG to be fragmented into its first product ion with m/z 168.2. Cutting or further fragmentation is on the C = O bond that causes 8-OHdG to be fragmented again into its product ion of m/z 140.1.

3.2 Verification method

The equation of straight line with R^2 = 0.9985 is obtained. Limit of Detection (LOD) is the smallest quantity of analytical concentration detectable from an analytical method while Limit of Quantification (LOQ) is the smallest accurate and meticulous quantity of the smallest calculated (quantified) concentration. The LOD and LOQ calculations were performed on the basis of a standard 8-OHdG standard calculation which had previously been performed for linearity determination, determined from the standard 8-OHdG calibration curve to the ratio of chromatogram area. From the calculation of statistics, obtained LOD value is 1,315 ppb and LOQ value is 4.384 ppb.

3.3 Analysis of 8-Hydroxy-2'-Deoxyguanosine in urine samples

3.3.1 Urine sampling and urine sample pre-treatment

This research has also gone through protocol study so that it can pass the ethical review through Medical Research Ethics Commission of Faculty of Medicine, University of Indonesia Jakarta based on letter number 0386/UN2.F1/ETIK/2018 and protocol number 18-03-0321.

Each week each rat was taken urine according to the method in point 2.2.3. Rats are placed in a metabolic cage for their urine shelter. For urine, the volume varies between 1 and 5 ml.

Before the sample is analyzed by LC–MS / MS instrument, the sample is passed first in the SPE column. SPE with column C18 allows to remove substances that interfere in the urine. The SPE method also shows considerable reproducibility and accuracy [16]. Pre-treatment of samples with SPE is necessary because if not treated first, it may interfere with measurements on LC–MS/MS instruments.

3.3.2 Effect of BPA on formation of DNA adduct 8-OHdG

After an 8-OHdG analysis was performed on the rats' urine samples of group B (rats given BPA exposure), a chromatogram was obtained with results as in **Figure 5**. 8-OHdG was detected at retention time of 0.773 minutes.

BPA exposure in rats has an effect that may lead to the formation of DNA adduct 8-OHdG. As shown in **Figure 6**, the 8-OHdG levels in rats exposed to BPA were greater than controls. Levels of 8-OHdG in rats given exposure to BPA also increased from exposure time of 1st to 4th week is from 27.041 ng/mL up to 31.220 ng/mL.

In this condition, the concentration of 8-OHdG is also above the LOD value. This is sufficient to prove that 8-OHdG as biomarker of DNA damage [17] can be formed and detected due to in vivo BPA exposure.

The results of this study indicate that BPA can increase the formation of hydroxyl radicals, which can bind to DNA to form 8-OHdG. The mechanism that causes BPA to lead to the formation of 8-OHdG is due to the fact that BPA can covalently induce the formation of ROS that can bind to DNA in vivo [18]. Metabolic conversion of BPA to DNA is catalyzed by cytochrome P450 in the liver to form 5-hydroxybisphenol [19]. Hydroxybisphenol is a catecholestrogen compound that is capable of redox cycling. Hydroxybisphenol is further oxidized to semiquinone, then the semiquinone will be further oxidized to 4,5-Bisphenol-O-quinone [18]. The catechol-o-quinone is capable of redox cycling with generation of oxidative

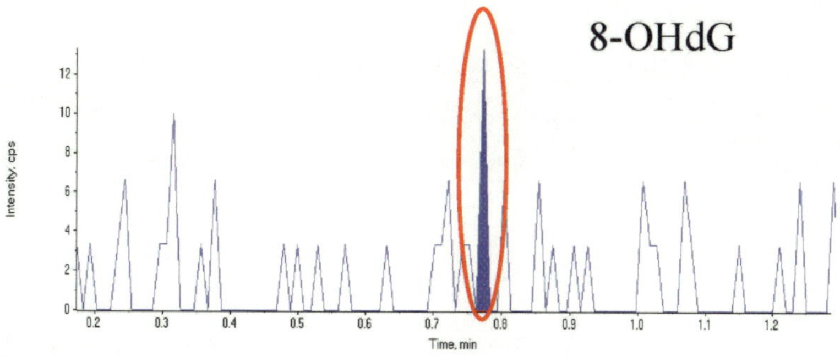

Figure 5.
Chromatogram of rats' urine samples given BPA exposure.

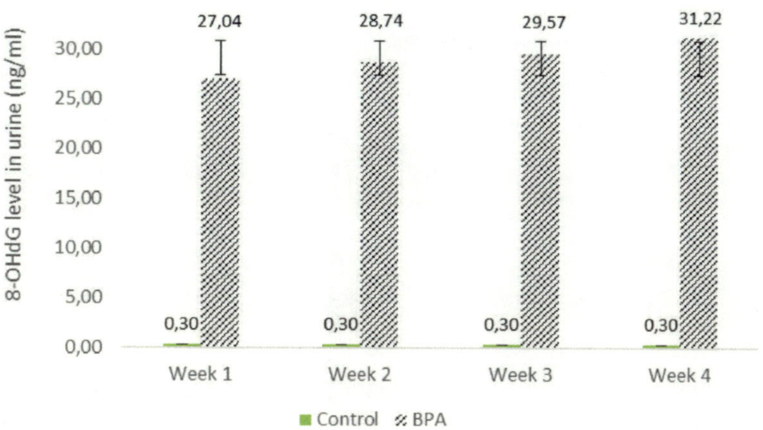

Figure 6.
The comparison graph of 8-OHdG concentrations between control rats and rats given BPA exposure.

stress (OS) and reactive oxygen species (ROS). o-Quinones are highly electron affinic with potential reduction that permit electron transfer (ET) under physiological conditions. Large quantities of ROS are sufficient to generate catalytically by small amounts of o-Quinones. There is extensive evidence for generation of ROS, which include ET by o-quinone as a plausible source. There are numerous reports on toxicity to body constituents by BPA [20]. The metabolic reaction was illustrated in **Figure 7**.

3.3.3 Effect of Ni (II) on formation of DNA adduct 8-OHdG

After an 8-OHdG analysis was performed on the rats' urine samples of group C (rats given exposure to BPA and Ni (II) metals), a chromatogram was obtained with results as in **Figure 8**. 8-OHdG in rats' urine samples exposed to BPA and Ni (II) metals were detected at retention time of 0.733 min.

Exposure to BPA and Ni (II) metals may also have an effect that may lead to the formation of an 8-OHdG DNA adduct. As shown in **Figure 9**, 8-OHdG levels in mice exposed to BPA and Ni (II) metals were greater than those of controls.

The 8-OHdG concentration in mice given exposure to BPA and Ni (II) at a dosage of 0.1 μg/kg bw also increased from exposure time of 1st to 4th week ie from 26.185 ng/mL to 28.696 ng/mL. In this condition, the concentration of 8-OHdG is also above the LOD value. This is sufficient to prove that 8-OHdG can be formed and detected due to exposure to BPA and metal Ni (II) in vivo.

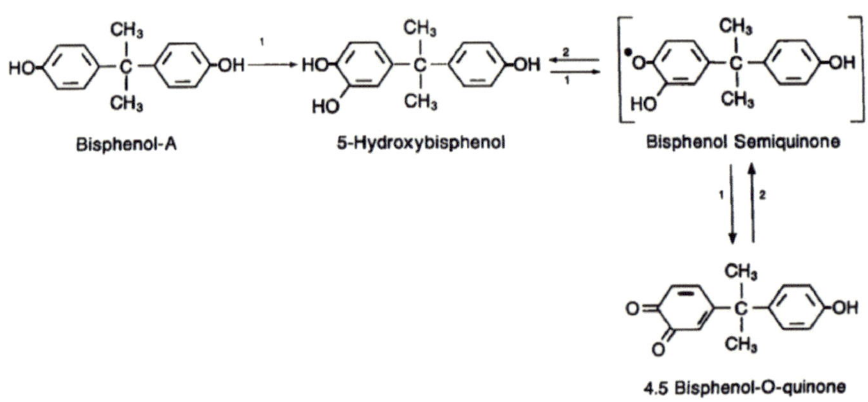

Figure 7.
Possible BPA mechanism in the human body (reprocessed). 1: Cytochrome P450; 2: Cytochrome P450 reductase. (Source: Atkinson and Roy [18]).

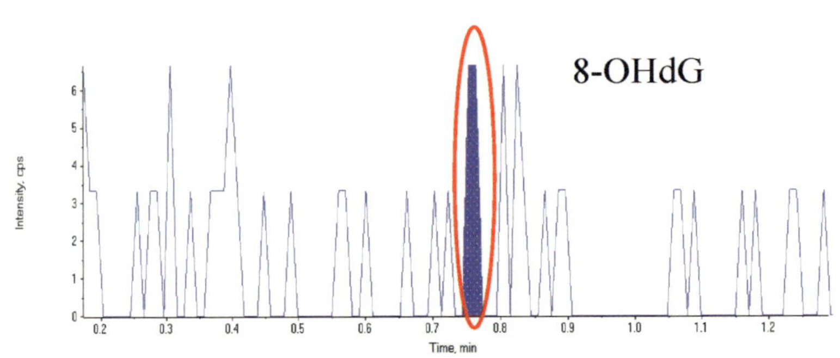

Figure 8.
Chromatogram of mouse urine samples given exposure to BPA and Ni (II).

One of the harmful effects of the nickel mechanism in the body is to induce the formation of ROS and increase lipid peroxidation in the cells [21]. Given that nickel is not an essential element for humans, it is not yet clear how nickel compounds go through the metabolic phase.

However, the resulting 8-OHdG levels of rats given exposure to BPA and Ni (II) were smaller than the 8-OHdG levels produced by rats given BPA exposure alone. The results can be seen in **Figure 10**.

This may be due to metabolic differences between rats and also because the doses given to mice are too small. A dose of 0.1 μg/kg bb resulted in an 8-OHdG increase each week in rats, but the levels remained smaller than the 8-OHdG levels obtained from rats given BPA exposure.

Oxidative stress of DNA of transition metals can possibly occurred due to the presence of free radicals produced by Fenton or Fenton-like reaction [22]. The major form of free radicals are hydroxyl radicals [17]. Nickel (II) at the excessive

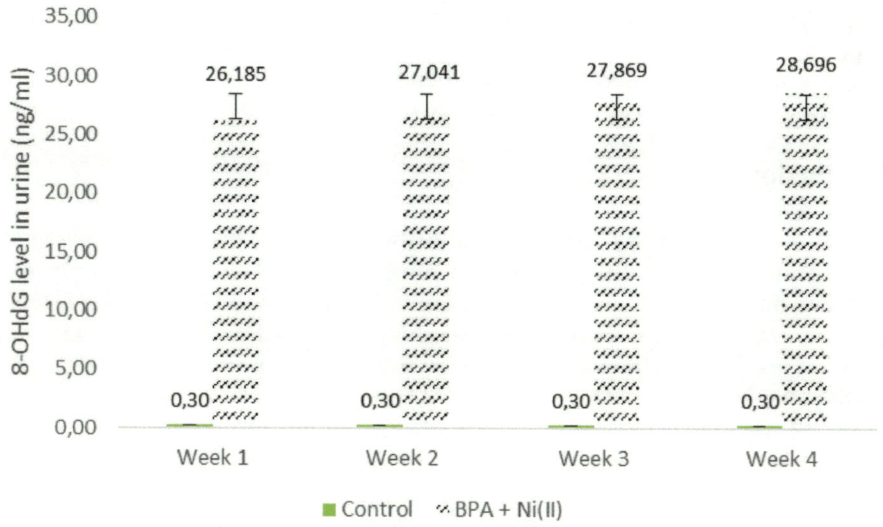

Figure 9.
The comparison graph of 8-OHdG concentrations in control and mouse rats given exposure to BPA and Ni (II).

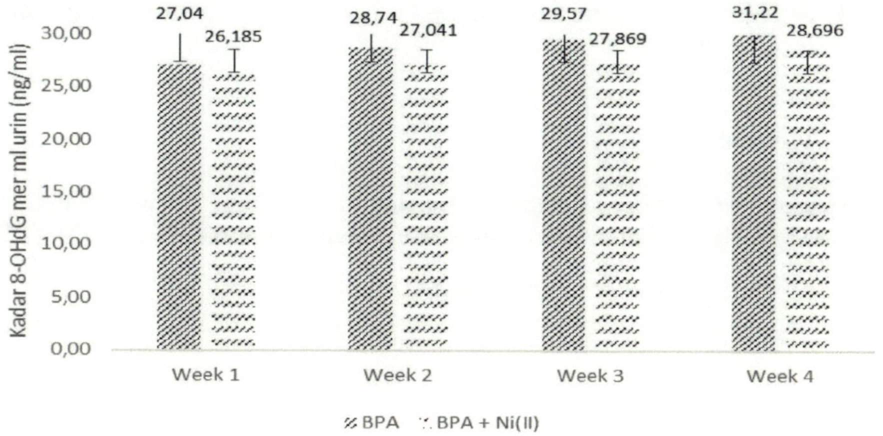

Figure 10.
Graph of comparison of 8-OHdG levels in rats given exposure to BPA and rats given exposure to BPA and Ni (II).

levels has a role in Fenton-like reaction to the formation of free radicals. Nickel (II) exposure in rats can cause a significant increase in lipid peroxidation, and a decrease of antioxidant enzymes such as superoxide dismutase (SOD), catalase (CAT), and glutathione peroxidase (GSH) [23].

Ni^{2+} is the largest nickel ionic species in the cell. There is the possibility of a Fenton-like reaction with nickel but only with the Ni^{2+} interaction with certain ligands, such as Gli-Gli-His (Glycyl-Glycyl-Histidin) or imidazole nitrogen from histidine [24]. The binding of Ni^{2+} to these ligands eliminates the oxidation potential of Ni^{2+} in which hydrogen peroxide can catalyze the oxidation of nickel to a higher oxidation state. This reaction produces a radical but the reaction depends on the binding of Ni^{2+} with certain ligands [25]. Thus, although nickel can produce oxidative stress in cells and oxidize the DNA bases, certain nickel compounds with carcinogenic potentials exhibit weak mutagenic activity in some mutation tests. However, chromosomal damage that causes mutations of a detectable gene produced by some nickel compounds may contribute to its carcinogenesis properties [26]. One interesting feature of the nickel compound is its synergistic nature with other compounds or agents that can cause cancer by its mutagenic mechanism. For example, synergic nickel with benzo [a]pirene, UV, and radiation [11]. It can also explain the absence of synergistic effects between BPA and Ni (II).

4. Conclusions

DNA adduct 8-Hydroxy-2'-Deoxyguanosine (8-OHdG) on urine sample of rats as a biomarker of DNA damage from BPA compounds and Ni (II) metals exposure, was formed and achieved the detection limit value. Levels of DNA adduct 8-OHdG in Sprague–Dawley rats after BPA/BPA and Ni (II) exposure was higher than levels of 8-OHdG in Sprague–Dawley control rats. It was also found that there was an increase in levels of DNA adduct 8-OHdG in Sprague–Dawley rats exposed to BPA and BPA-Ni (II) metals from first week exposure time until fourth week of exposure time (28 days). However, levels of 8-OHdG in rats exposed by BPA-Ni (II) is less than levels of 8-OHdG in rats exposed by BPA only. It can caused by the doses of BPA-Ni (II) metals administered to rats were in a non-excessive state, therefore the synergic effect of two toxic substances in the formation of 8-OHdG has not already been seen. There is possibility of the role of o-Quinones in metabolic cycle of BPA administered the increases of hydroxyl radical levels. And the role of Fenton-like reaction might give synergistic effect in the formation of hydroxyl radicals at the excessive level of Ni(II).

Acknowledgements

The authors would like to thank Universitas Indonesia for funding this research through PITTA Grant Universitas Indonesia 2018 with contract number 2242/UN2.R3.1/HKP.05.00/2018.

DOI: http://dx.doi.org/10.5772/intechopen.99432

Author details

Budiawan*, Intan Cahaya Dani, Chrissy Fransisca Olivyana Rugian and Sri Handayani
Faculty of Mathematics and Natural Science, Department of Chemistry, Universitas Indonesia, Depok, Indonesia

*Address all correspondence to: dr.budiawan@sci.ui.ac.id

References

[1] Wang, Z., Liu, H. and Liu, S. (2016). Low-Dose BisphenolA Exposure: A Seemingly Instigating Carcinogenic Effect on Breast Cancer. Advanced Science, 4(2), p.1600248.

[2] Olea, N., Pulgar, R., Perez, P., Olea-Serrano, F., Rivas, A., Novillo-Fertrell, A., Pedraza, V., Soto, A. and Sonnenschein, C. (1996). Estrogenicity of Resin-Based Composites and Sealants Used in Dentistry. Environmental Health Perspectives, 104(3), p.298.

[3] Vandenberg LN, Colborn T, Hayes TB, Heindel JJ, Jacobs Jr DR, Lee DH, et al. Hormones and endocrine-disrupting chemicals: low-dose effects and nonmonotonic dose responses. (2012). Endocr Rev, 33:378-455.

[4] Vinas R, Jeng YJ, Watson CS. Non-genomic effects of xenoestrogen mixtures. (2012). Int J Environ Res Public Health 9:2694-2714.

[5] Tiwari, D., Vanage, G. Bisphenol A Induces Oxidative Stress in Bone Marrow Cells, Lymphocytes, and Reproductive Organs of Holtzman Rats. (2017). International Journal of Toxicology, 36(2) 142-152.

[6] Hasselberg L, Meier S, Svardal A. (2004). Effects of alkylphenols on redox status in first spawning Atlantic cod (Gadus morhua). Aquat Toxicol.69(1): 95-105.

[7] Zhao, J., Magaya, R., Zou, B., Shi, H., Yu, H., Yue, X., Liu, K., Lin, X., Xu, J., Yang, C. and Wu, A. (2008). Acute toxicity of nickel nanoparticles in rats after intravenous injection. International Journal of Nanomedicine, p.1393.

[8] International Agency for Research on Cancer (IARC). (1990). IARC Summary & Evaluation, Volume 49. Inchem.org. N.p., 1990.

[9] Lloyd, D., Carmichael, P. and Phillips, D. (1998). Comparison of the Formation of 8-Hydroxy-2'-deoxyguanosine and Single- and Double-Strand Breaks in DNA Mediated by Fenton Reactions. Chemical Research in Toxicology, 11(5), pp.420-427.

[10] Frenkel, K. (1992). Carcinogen-mediated oxidant formation and oxidative DNA damage. Pharmacology & Therapeutics, 53(1), pp.127-166.

[11] Fraga CG, Shigenaga MK, Park JW, Degan P, Ames BN. Oxidative damage to DNA during aging: 8-hydroxy-20-deoxyguanosine in rat organ DNA and urine. Proc Natl Acad Sci. 1990;87(12): 4533-4537.

[12] Cheng KC, Cahill DS, Kasai H, Nishimura S, Loeb LA. 8-Hydroxyguanine, an abundant form of oxidative DNA damage, causes G-T and A-C substitutions. J Biol Chem. 1992;267(1): 166-172.

[13] Lu AL, Li X, Gu Y, Wright PM, Chang DY. Repair of oxidative DNA damage: mechanisms and functions. Cell Biochem Biophys.2001;35(2): 41-170.

[14] Guo, C., Li, X., Wang, R., Yu, J., Ye, M., Mao, L., Zhang, S. and Zheng, S. (2016). Association between Oxidative DNA Damage and Risk of Colorectal Cancer: Sensitive Determination of Urinary 8-Hydroxy-2′-deoxyguanosine by UPLC-MS/MS Analysis. Scientific Reports, 6(1).

[15] Moriwaki, Hiroshi. (2000). Determination Of 8-Hydroxy-2'-Deoxyguanosine In Urine By Liquid Chromatography-Electrospray Ionization-Mass Spectrometry. Analytical Sciences 16.2.105-106.

[16] Koide, Satoshi et al. (2010). Determination Of Human Serum

8-Hydroxy-2′-Deoxyguanosine (8-Ohdg) By HPLC-ECD Combined With Solid Phase Extraction (SPE). Journal of Chromatography B 878.23. 2163-2167. Web.

[17] Valavanidis, A., Vlachogianni, T., Flotakis, C., 2009, 8-hydroxy-2'-deoxyguanosine (8-OHdG):A Critical Biomarker of Oxidative Stress and Carcinogenesis. Journal of Environmental Science and Health Part C, 27:120-139, 2009.

[18] Atkinson, Alfonza, and Deodutta Roy. (1995) "In Vivo DNA Adduct Formation by BisphenolA. Environmental and Molecular Mutagenesis, vol. 26, no. 1, pp. 60-66., doi:10.1002/em.2850260109.

[19] Elsby R, Maggs JL, Ashby J, Park BK (2001) Comparison of the modulatory effects of human and rat liver microsomal metabolism on the estrogenicity of bisphenol A: implications for extrapolation to humans. J Pharmacol Exp Ther 297 (1): 103-113. PubMed: 11259533.

[20] Kovacic, Peter. (2010). How safe is bisphenol A? Fundamentals of toxicity: Metabolism, electron transfer and oxidative stress. Medical hypotheses. 75. 1-4.

[21] Lambade, P.S. et al. (2015). Clinicopathological Studies Of Experimentally Induced Nickel Chloride In Wistar Rats (RattusNorvegicus)." Indian Journal of Veterinary Pathology 39.1. 41.

[22] Klein, C., Costa, M., 2007, Handbook on the Toxicology of Metals (3rd ed.), ed. Nordberg, G. F., Fowler, B., A., Nordberg, M., and Friberg, L. T., Elsevier Academic Press, Oxford, p.743.

[23] Das, K. K., Das, S. N., Dhundasi, S. A. (2008). Nickel, its adverse health effects & oxidative stress. Indian J Med Res 128, October 2008, pp 412-425.

[24] Zalups, Rudolfs K, and Donald James Koropatnick. (2000). Molecular Biology And Toxicology Of Metals. London: Taylor & Francis, 2000. Print.

[25] Klein, Catherine B. et al. (1991). "The Role Of Nickel And Nickel-Mediated Reactive Oxygen Species In The Mechanism Of Nickel Carcinogenesis." Environmental Health Perspectives 102: 281. Web.

[26] Costa, M. (1991). Molecular Mechanisms Of Nickel Carcinogenesis. Annual Review of Pharmacology and Toxicology 31.1: 321-337. Web

Chapter 2

Interaction of Bisphenol A with G Protein: Coupled Receptors - New Paradigms in Breast Cancer

Luis Molina, Carlos D. Figueroa and Pamela Ehrenfeld

Abstract

The massive use of bisphenols, actually bisphenol A, in consumer products and food packaging has been associated with certain hazardous conditions for human health, which include their interactions with a family of specific membrane receptors and their effects as endocrine disruptors related to breast cancer. For this reason, bisphenol A was removed from many products, but it has been replaced by structural analogs whose pathways of action and metabolic effects are so far partially unknown. This chapter emphasizes the discovery of bisphenols, their uses in human life, and their impact on health population by focusing on breast cancer. Regarding their mechanisms of action, we have focused on the signaling routes activated by bisphenols following their binding to G protein–coupled receptors.

Keywords: estrogen, bisphenols, GPCRs, breast cancer, endocrine disruptors, G protein-coupled estrogen receptor 1 (GPER-1), angiotensin receptors (AT), adrenergic receptors (AR), chemokine receptors

1. Introduction

Significant evidence suggests that endocrine disruption is attributable not only to pharmaceutical products or rare contaminants, but also to exogenous chemical compounds ubiquitously found in everyday life of the modern world. Endocrine-disrupting chemicals (EDCs) enter the human body where they act similarly to endogenous hormones, altering endocrine homeostasis and causing adverse effects on human health [1–7]. Interestingly, the US Food and Drug Administration identified more than 1800 chemical disruptors of endocrine pathways involving estrogen, androgen, and thyroid hormones [8]. EDCs have been related to the development of disorders such as adulthood diabetes, poor semen quality, polycystic ovary syndrome, neurodegenerative disorders, and cancer [1, 8]. Changes in the physiological levels of hormones circulating in the human body may be involved in the high incidence of tumors of the reproductive system in both men and women [8]. Indeed, breast cancer is the most common cancer diagnosed in women worldwide that has been associated in a small percentage with genetic predisposition (*BRCA1* and *BRCA2* mutations) whereas the majority of breast tumors have been categorized as sporadic breast cancer [9]. In fact, lifestyle factors such as smoking, alcohol consumption, sedentary lifestyle, and obesity have been related to the development of the disease. However, an increasing body of evidence suggests that etiology for breast cancer may be related at least in part to exposure to chemicals of some kind. Indeed, recent studies show that environmental pollutants could also play a role in the pathogenesis and progression of breast cancer. Evidence from epidemiological studies and basic science using *in vitro* and *in vivo* models suggests that exposure to EDCs may be positively correlated with breast cancer development, particularly when the exposure occurred during critical stages of human life. The list of suspected environmental pollutants having a role in breast cancer is extensive and includes polychlorides, biphenyl ethers, phthalates, triclosan, octylphenol, dichlorodiphenyltrichloroethane, and bisphenols (BPs). Bisphenol A (BPA), or 4,40-dihydroxy-2,2-diphenylpropane, is one of the main compounds of this class; BPA is an organic synthetic plastic monomer that was first synthesized in the 1890s as a synthetic estrogen and a key element in the manufacture of cans, reusable water bottles, and medical equipment. BPA regulates several processes, such as cell proliferation, migration, and apoptosis, leading to neoplastic changes due to its ability to mimic the actions of estrogen at multiple levels by activating both α and β estrogen receptors (ERα and ERβ). The effects of BPA on the reproductive system of rats were reported in the 1930s. Now, 91 years later, several studies performed in mice have demonstrated DNA damage, induction of oxidative stress, and epigenetic changes in oocytes [8]. BPA can induce various types of modifications in the reproductive system of men and women, supporting multiple oncogenic signaling routes such as STAT3, PI3K/Akt, and MAPK pathways [8]. Benign lesions that can progress to breast or ovarian cancer due to BPA depend on several molecular and epigenetic mechanisms that will determine whether the endocrine or the reproductive system is affected and will be reviewed in this chapter. Moreover, the effects of BPs on GPCRs associated with breast cancer development or progression are addressed.

2. Xenoestrogens derived from anthropogenic activity

2.1 Some historical aspects of bisphenol A and related compounds

In 1891 Aleksandr Dianin, a Russian chemist from Saint Petersburg, combined phenol with acetone in the presence of an acid catalyst, synthesizing for the first time the chemical substance called 4,40-dihydroxy-2,2-diphenylpropane [10], a molecule that was later recognized by the name of bisphenol A [11]. In 1936, the English scientists Dodds and Lawson reported that BPA exhibited important estrogenic properties inducing complete cornification in vaginal smears of ovariectomized rats treated with this compound [12]. In the 1940s, BPA was basically considered a synthetic estrogen and its potential carcinogenic properties in humans started to be studied [13, 14]. Therefore, BPA is one of the first compounds of anthropogenic origin in which an endocrine-disrupting activity has been verified.

Later in the 1950s, it was found that the reaction of BPA with phosgene generated a polycarbonate, unalterable over time, easy to mold, versatile, and transparent. Due to these multiple qualities, together with its chemical stability, the industry began to use it rapidly and massively to manufacture all types of plastic containers [2]. Currently, BPA has been used to produce various electronic and construction products, automotive parts, medical and clinical articles, toys for children, hygiene and personal care items, and storage products. In addition, it is used for the inner lining of metal cans for preservation of food and beverages [2]. For this reason, BPA is today one of the most used chemical products worldwide. Several studies have suggested that the greatest human exposure to BPA (>90%) is likely to occur through food contamination and, to a lesser extent, by dust ingestion and absorption through the skin or dental surgeries [8].

The proestrogenic activity of BPA resurfaced in the early 1990s when a team led by David Feldman identified through mass spectrometry the presence of this molecule in a growth medium of yeast (*Saccharomyces cerevisiae*) and even in the pure water contained in the autoclaved polycarbonate flasks [15]. In turn, one of the first effects of BPA was evaluated in breast cancer cells. Indeed, in estrogen-sensitive MCF-7 human breast cancer cells (ERα-positive cells), BPA induced a great expression of progesterone receptors and increased their proliferation rate [3, 15]. From this period to date, numerous investigations have reported the potential risk that continuous exposure to BPA implies for human and animal health and ecosystems [3]. This evidence has contributed to consider BPA as one of the main xenoestrogens of ubiquitous environmental distribution. In response to these effects, the industry has sought alternatives to traditional BPA, generating a variety of new bisphenols, such as bisphenol S (BPS), bisphenol AF (BPAF), bisphenol E (BPE), bisphenol B (BPB), and bisphenol F (BPF) among other phenolic molecules, some of which have also been related to estrogenic activity and are considered physiological disruptors of varying degrees in humans [3, 16].

2.2 Routes of BPA exposure and metabolism

The continuous presence of BPA in our environment suggests that several routes of exposure may exist. Oral ingestion seems to be the main route, given the storage of food and liquids in plastic containers that include BPA among its major constituents, which also diffuses into the environment after exposure to high temperatures or frequent washing. The US EPA has established a safe daily intake of 50 g BPA/kg of body weight per day based on the assumption that the main source of exposure to BPA is through food ingestion [17]. Not only in humans but also in primates, ingested BPA is rapidly absorbed (5–15 min later) by the intestinal wall and is transformed into BPA glucuronide following its first passage through the intestine and liver; in addition, a small fraction of BPA is also transformed into a sulfate conjugate [4, 16, 18, 19]. Conjugated forms of BPA are estimated to have no endocrine activity [19, 20]. In murine models, and after oral administration of nanomolar doses of BPA, oxidation products of this compound have been found, suggesting the formation of secondary metabolites with greater estrogenic activity than the parent molecule [5]. BPA has a half-life between 4 and 5 h, and most of the conjugated forms are finally excreted through the urine [4, 5, 16]. Inhalation seems to be another route of entry, inducing cough, bronchospasm, and asthmatic attacks; similarly, eye exposure may cause conjunctivitis, itching, and periorbital edema whereas skin contact usually produces localized redness and inflammation [19].

BPA has been detected in all biological fluids, including serum, urine, cerebrospinal fluid, and milk, in most of today's human populations. In fetal tissues, BPA has been found in concentrations similar to those present in maternal blood, showing that it can cross the transplacental barrier [19]. Furthermore, toxicological data indicates that human embryos and neonates, unlike adults, cannot conjugate BPA increasing its possibility to exert toxic effects [5]. Epidemiological and experimental studies suggest that embryonic exposure to BPA is in the long term related to the occurrence of a series of disorders, such as precocious puberty, infertility, metabolic disorders, and a series of hormone-dependent tumors, like breast cancer [1, 5, 17, 20, 21].

2.3 Pathophysiological effects of bisphenols: endocrine, metabolic, and carcinogenic disruptors

To date, only a few studies have explored the effects produced by exposure to BPs, mainly BPA, during intrauterine or postnatal life together with their effects on general human health. Multiple metabolic disorders, polycystic ovary syndrome, spontaneous abortion, infertility, endometrial hyperplasia, hormone-dependent tumors, immunity alterations, cardiovascular pathologies, neurodegenerative disorders and obesity have so far been reported among their deleterious effects on human health [1]. Dumitrascu et al. in 2019 [1] highlighted that women suffering from polycystic ovary syndrome exhibited higher circulating levels of BPA and testosterone than healthy women and that high androgen levels decreased BPA clearance. Furthermore, they pointed out that women with endometriosis showed high levels of BPA in serum, suggesting an association between this compound and the disease. It has also been suggested that patients with high urinary levels of BPA have a high probability of implantation failure during *in vitro* fertilization procedures. In young people, an early exposure to BPA has been associated with high percentage of body fat, elevated body mass index, and abdominal circumference and numerous neurological implications, such as anxious or depressive behavior, all conditions that have been suggested to increase the risk of developing cancer. Comparative studies between BPA and its analogs (BPB, BPF, and BPS) show that they have toxic effects on the testes and spermatogenesis that are mediated by an increase in the levels of oxidative stress and a decrease in the levels of enzymes with antioxidant activity [22]; some of them may also have a neuroendocrine disrupting activity [6] (see **Figure 1**). Examples of neurobehavioral disorders associated with BPA in different experimental models (rodents, zebrafish, and *Caenorhabditis elegans*) range from cognitive deficit, increased anxiety, socio-sexual deficiencies to hyperactivity or autism spectrum disorders. It is postulated that neurological effects may be due to the weak estrogenic effect of BPA or its analogs by binding to estrogen receptors in different areas of the brain [6, 23].

With regard to the risk of developing malignant neoplasms, the greatest association has been observed with breast, ovarian, and prostate cancer though the studies have not been conclusive [1]. To overcome the effects of BPA associated with an increased public concern about the risk of developing endocrine-related cancer due to exposure to BPA [24], the industry has replaced it with analogs such as BPS, BPB, BPF, or BPAF, which are now parts of products labeled as BPA-free [25]. Nevertheless, *in vitro* assays have demonstrated that BPAF has a stronger binding affinity for estrogen receptors when compared with BPA [26].

Likewise, recent studies have shown that both BPA and BPS can contribute to breast cancer malignancy by disrupting the organization of acinar structures and by affecting the normal development of the mammary gland [9]. To date, the effects of BPA in eukaryotic cells have been reported to be mediated primarily by steroid receptors, including ERα and ERβ, estrogen-related receptors (ERR), androgen receptors (AR), and peroxisome proliferator-activated

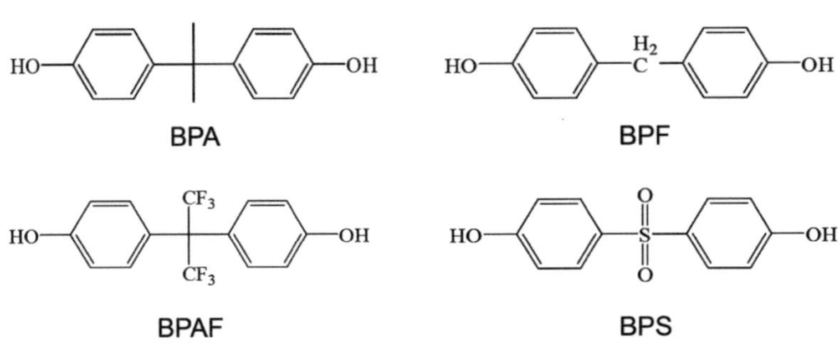

Figure 1.
Structure of main bisphenols produced by industrial activity. BPA, bisphenol A; BPF, bisphenol F; BPAF, bisphenol AF; BPS, bisphenol S.

receptors (PPAR) [24]. Other interactions include signaling by stimulation of angiotensin (AT), α-adrenergic (AR,) or chemokine (CXC) receptors.

3. Bisphenols and their role in breast cancer

Although BPA does not possess the potency of estrogen, it is ubiquitously distributed in nature and its resistance to enzymatic or chemical degradation makes it even more dangerous. Breast cancer has a high mortality in women in many countries, and approximately 10% of these tumors are due to genetic influence whereas 90% are related to lifestyle or associated with negative elements present in the surrounding environment [1]. The most harmful effects attributed to EDCs would occur during breast development when this tissue is more susceptible to developing atypical differentiation. *In vivo* studies show that prolonged exposure (60 days) of breast cells to 400 μg of BPA/kg of body weight induces an increase in the density of mammary buds [27], in cell proliferation, and in the levels of oxidative stress without significant differences in the expression of estrogen receptors [1, 27, 28]. Previous studies have demonstrated that women who exhibit mutations in the tumor suppressor genes *BRCA1* and *BRCA2* in mammary gland cells have a greater risk of developing breast cancer and also a high susceptibility to the negative effects of environmental BPA [1, 27, 29]. In normal or cancerous adult breast tissue, BPA has been associated with an increased proliferation rate and with the induction of chemoresistance in ERα-positive cells [1, 30, 31]. BPA can also modify DNA repair, inactivate p53, and induce changes in genes associated with apoptosis to stop cell death through DNA methylation. By activating vascular endothelial growth factor, BPA can increase angiogenesis in breast tumors [32] and at the same time activate the MAPK and STAT pathways to modulate the proliferation kinetics of human mammary epithelial cells [1, 33].

Breast cell cultures developed in a 3D fashion are one of the most widely used models to gain a better understanding of the role of bisphenols in breast cancer. Using this approach and MCF-12A cells, which exhibit a typical luminal epithelial morphology, it was observed that low doses of BPA and BPS generated a disruption in the normal organization of the mammary acinus and promoted cell invasion [9]. Interestingly, mammospheres of MCF-7 cells (ERα-positive cell line) treated with 10 nM BPA displayed high expression of aldehyde dehydrogenase 1, a marker of breast stem cells, and SOX-2, a key transcription factor for cell pluripotentiality and self-renewal. That effects were not observed when MDA-MB-231 (ERα-negative cell line) was used instead of MCF-7 cells, suggesting that the receptors through which BPA modulates its signaling exhibit a different expression pattern in this kind of cancer, highlighting the implications of the heterogenicity of tumor mammary tissue when evaluating the effects of EDCs [34].

Evidence suggests that BPA may play an important role in the lifecycle and carcinogenesis of mammary epithelial cells and challenge us to continue studying its role in the origin and progression of breast cancer. One approach is to determine the relationship between BPA and G protein–coupled receptors (GPCRs) signaling, considering the recent evidence of the role of GPER-1 in breast cancer progression. Interestingly, approximately 20% of human neoplasms are related to some alteration in GPCRs [35]. The first relationship of GPCRs with tumorigenesis dates back to the 1980s, when a novel proto-oncogene called *MAS1* was described together with its ability to encode a hydrophobic protein of 325 amino acids with seven transmembrane domains. Today, it is known that the *MAS1* proto-oncogene generates a GPCR that binds to angiotensin (1–7), a metabolite of angiotensin II [35]; therefore, MAS1 receptor is part of the signaling cascade that supports the endocrine activity of the renin-angiotensin-aldosterone system (RAS), which regulates the proliferative or antiproliferative effects produced by hormones participating in the RAS pathway [36]. At present, it has been shown that components of RAS are expressed in various types of cancer, including breast cancer [37]. Additionally, several members of the large family of GPCRs have been identified as promoters of carcinogenesis, interacting directly or indirectly with BPA and other phenolic compounds to generate disruptive effects not only during adulthood but also during intrauterine and early postnatal life.

4. Implications of bisphenols on GPCRs signaling in breast cancer: GPER-1, angiotensin, CXC, and α-adrenergic receptors

4.1 General characteristics of GPCRs

The ability to receive and transmit a variety of external and internal signals is a fundamental feature to coordinate morphological and functional activities of multicellular organisms. The notion that receptive structures and substances mediate cellular responses was envisioned in 1897 by Paul Ehrlich with his "side chain" theory [38] and formulated more directly in 1905 by John Newport Langley [39]. However, at that time, the techniques to verify this hypothesis did not exist. It was not until the 1970s that Lefkowitz, using (−) [^{3}H] alprenolol, a potent β-adrenergic antagonist, achieved the specific binding of this ligand to β-adrenergic receptors in frog red blood cells [40] and purified the β-adrenergic receptor (AR) by using affinity chromatography [41]. Since then, it has been demonstrated that the binding of a β-adrenergic agonist to its receptor leads to the activation of the heterotrimeric G protein with the subsequent production of cAMP [42]. The structure of this receptor was later investigated in more detail by Kobilka employing X-ray crystallography who found a surprising homology of β-adrenergic receptor with the previously described rhodopsin receptor [43, 44]. Elucidation of the structural and functional features of the β-adrenergic receptor, including its crystallization, constitutes one of the most relevant scientific milestones in recent times on the knowledge of GPCRs.

Currently, technical advances in molecular biology have made it possible to determine the genetic code of numerous receptor proteins, identifying their amino acidic sequence and allowing interesting evolutionary relationships. GPCRs represent approximately 4% of all genes encoded by the human genome, generating between 650 and 800 different types of GPCRs, constituting the most numerous family of membrane receptors, regulating a large number of physiological and pathological processes [39]. It is estimated that 60% of all commercially available drugs target at least one particular GPCR [45].

The most accepted classification of GPCRs is supported by the International Union of Basic and Clinical Pharmacology (IUPHAR), which based on structural and phylogenetic criteria has grouped them into the families of rhodopsin (family A), secretin (family B), and glutamate (family C) and into the adhesion receptor or frizzled/taste2 families [46]. The structural characteristics and the degree of homology between the different families make it possible to determine that all GPCRs in humans derive from a single common ancestor [46, 47]. GPCRs are characterized by having seven transmembrane helices, with an amino-terminal end located extracellularly and a carboxy-terminal end located toward the interior of the cell, in the vicinity of which the interaction with the heterotrimeric G protein occurs, promoting intracellular signaling events once the receptor is activated by its corresponding agonist [46]. It is estimated that GPCRs arose about 1200 million years ago, during the evolutionary separation of alveolates (organisms that do not have GPCRs in their genome) from fungi and plants (organisms that do present some types of GPCRs) [47, 48]. More than 80% of all GPCRs belong to the rhodopsin family, characterized by highly conserved motifs and significant structural and functional diversity [46, 47].

GPCRs are integral proteins of the plasma membrane that interact with a large number and variety of signals such as photons, ions, neurotransmitters, peptides, and hormones of different chemical nature [49]. Among the physiological responses triggered by GPCRs are the regulation of cell survival, motility, and cell proliferation [47]. It has been shown that in addition to classical nuclear ERα and ERβ receptors, endogenous estrogens can exert their biological activity by binding to cell membrane-sited receptors, particularly some of the large family of GPCRs [50, 51].

4.2 Bisphenols and their effects beyond nuclear estrogen receptors

As mentioned before, BPA is one of the most studied xenoestrogens, initially developed as estrogen and now produced in large quantities and added to many consumer products such as coatings for cans, dental fillings, plastic bottles, feeding bottles, and some medical devices, causing ubiquitous human exposure. Indeed, more than 1 mg/kg of BPA has been detected in some foods, such as vegetables, probably due to leaks from plastic irrigation devices [24].

It is estimated that approximately 70% of breast carcinomas depend on estrogen and consequently are clinically classified as "hormone-sensitive breast cancer" or ERα-positive tumors. Interestingly, numerous reports indicate that xenoestrogens (chemicals that induce estrogen or antiestrogen responses) can disrupt normal estrogen-dependent signaling. Among the main xenoestrogens, BPA and some of the newly derived bisphenols stand out for their industrial origin and frequent occurrence in our "modern" society and ecosystems, generating a series of alterations in human beings and the environment. With no doubt, BPA is so far one of the most studied xenoestrogens though 17β-estradiol is the most potent form of estrogen when compared with BPA or other bisphenols [1, 50]. In men, estrogens favor serum levels of HDL cholesterol (high-density lipoproteins) to improve the cardiovascular condition and maintain bone mass and sperm maturation. In women, estrogens have strong effects on the female reproductive organs, including the breast, uterus, and menstrual cycle regulation. Moreover, altered estrogen balance is implicated in the pathophysiology of breast, ovarian, colorectal, prostate, and endometrial cancer. Similarly, estrogen unbalance has been implicated in metabolic, autoimmune, cardiovascular, neurodegenerative, and mood disorders [51].

BPA has long-term disruptive effects, even when contact has occurred during prenatal development. Intrauterine BPA exposure in pregnant Wistar rats alters the histoarchitecture of the mammary gland by increasing angiogenesis in female offsprings at postnatal day 50 or 110 [52]. Other studies, also using a murine model, indicate that prenatal exposure to BPA or its analogs, BPS and BPAF, induces accelerated development of the mammary gland, generating in the long term an increased susceptibility to spontaneous preneoplastic lesions, characterized by lobuloalveolar hyperplasia and perivascular inflammation [53].

As expected, the effects of BPA or other bisphenols have already been validated by studying their genomic activities on the pathways of nuclear estrogen receptors and it is only in the last years that the impact on GPCRs such as GPER-1, angiotensin, chemokines, and adrenergic receptors, as alternative estrogen-binding molecules, has begun to be elucidated [54]. Here, we present some evidence about interactions between BPs, GPCRs, breast cancer, and cancer progression.

4.3 G protein: coupled estrogen receptor 1 (GPER-1)

Since the discovery of nuclear ERα by Jensen, the binding of estradiol to cell surface receptors was considered highly unlikely [50]. However, a series of investigations that demonstrated increased levels of cAMP shortly after estrogen stimulation, as well as increased cell proliferation of ERα-deficient cells following stimulation with 17β-estradiol, suggested the presence of a membrane-located receptor that was interacting functionally with estrogen [50, 55]. In 2002, the activity of a membrane estrogen receptor, provisionally called "ER-X," was revealed, though its structure was not investigated [56]. Additionally, a glutamate receptor of the groups I and II sensitive to estrogen, whose activity was independent of Erα, was reported [57]. Given this background, several groups investigated an orphan membrane receptor called GPR30 (G protein-coupled receptor 30), described in 1997 by Carmeci et al., [58] which was strongly expressed in estrogen-sensitive breast cancer cells. In 2005, Thomas et al. demonstrated the specific binding of estrogen to GPR30 in SKBR3 breast cancer cells, a cell type that expresses GPR30 but not nuclear estrogen receptors [59]. In addition, Revankar et al. reported the localization of GPR30 in the endoplasmic reticulum and that its binding to estrogen increased intracellular calcium levels [60]. Subsequently, several groups, including ours, have described that GPR30 is primarily sited in the plasma membrane of breast cancer cells [50, 61]. Due to the ability of GPR30 to bind to estrogen, it was renamed as GPER-1 (G protein-coupled estrogen receptor 1) [61], a protein of 375 amino acids encoded by a gene located in chromosome 7p22.3 [61, 62]. GPER-1 activation triggers a non-genomic or "fast" intracellular signaling cascade characterized by cAMP production and increased intracellular calcium levels [63, 64], Src activation through Gβγ, with subsequent release of HB-EGF (heparin-binding EGF-like growth factor) and transactivation of EGFR (epidermal growth factor receptor) [61]. In addition, the activation of phospholipase C and cFos and several kinases such as ERK1/2 MAPK, PI3K (phosphoinositol 3-kinase), and Akt has also been described [50, 61, 63, 64].

In female GPER-1 null mice, an alteration of glucose homeostasis has been observed associated with a low release of insulin, reduced bone growth, and increased blood pressure [65] whereas male knock-out mice suffer deterioration of the cardiac function [66]. Furthermore, GPER-1 also modulates the immune system, inducing apoptosis of T cells and inhibiting the inflammatory process [67]. In summary, GPER-1 promotes a series of key biological functions attributed exclusively to nuclear α and β receptors in reproductive tissues, the cardiovascular system, the immune system, and the nervous system, among others [61]. GPER-1 has been linked to regulation of growth, migration, and survival of cancer cells [68] since it is expressed in ERα-positive and -negative breast tumors and their corresponding human breast cancer cell lines [50]. Clinical investigations have shown that patients with GPER-1 positive breast tumors and four to six months of tamoxifen treatment developed resistance to therapy and suffered an increase in breast tumor mass and reduced survival [68–70]. GPER-1 activation also produces an increase in the number of breast cancer stem cells (CSCs) by activating the TAZ protein (transcriptional coactivator with PDZ-binding motif), one of the components of the Hippo signaling pathway [71]. The ability to reprogram CSCs is also attributed to elevated TAZ in breast cancer [72]. A recent investigation using tumor cells isolated from ERα/PR-positive breast tumors showed that silencing of GPER-1 generated, *in vitro* and *in vivo*, mammospheres with a reduced population of CSCs [73]. By comparison, the activation of GPER-1 by estrogen or tamoxifen induced the phosphorylation of PKA, stimulating the growth of malignant cells, and the activation of BAD-Ser118, an event related to an increase in the activation of glucokinase with the consequent production of ATP in the mitochondria, which in turn may promote the maintenance and proliferation of CSCs [73]. Recently, we have reported that continuous exposure of MCF-7 cells (ERα/GPER-1-positive) to tamoxifen significantly increased intracellular calcium mobilization and cell proliferation through GPER-1 overexpression [64]. In addition, tamoxifen, estrogen, and the synthetic GPER-1 agonist, G1, have been shown to promote cell proliferation and cell cycle progression of cancer-associated fibroblasts (CAF) [74].

In general, xenoestrogens have been shown to have similar binding affinities for ERα, ERβ, and GPER-1. Interestingly, the phytoestrogen genistein and BPA have high affinity for GPER-1 [75]. It has been shown that nanomolar concentrations of BPA stimulate the proliferation of TM4 mouse Sertoli cells. Exposure of TM4 cells to ICI 182,780 or G15 (a GPER-1 antagonist) abolished the proliferative response promoted by BPA, pointing out a strong dependence from ERα/ERβ and GPER-1 [76]. In addition, it has been shown that BPA can produce a hypothalamic disrupting effect, particularly on the gonadotropin-releasing hormone (GnRH) release axis and, therefore, on the reproductive cycle in humans [77]. Moreover, nanomolar concentrations of BPA induce through GPER-1 and αvβ3 integrin, which acts as a vitronectin receptor, the proliferation of male germ cells [78].

A study using triple-negative breast cancer cells (TNBC) showed that BPS trigger cancer cells migration, through activation of the GPER/Hippo-YAP signaling pathway. The dephosphorylation of YAP (yes-associated protein) promotes its accumulation in the nucleus, upregulating *CTGF* and *ANKRD1* genes. GPER/Yap inhibition reduces triple-negative breast cancer cells' migration promoted by BPS [79]. In addition, nanomolar concentrations of BPAF and BPB have been shown to exert higher estrogenic effects than BPA on SKBR3 breast cancer cells (GPER-1-positive/ERα-negative), by activating GPER-1 signaling pathways [54]. Similarly, bisphenols can also exert estrogenic effects via GPER-1 in ERα-positive breast cancer cells. Thus, BPAF triggers intracellular calcium mobilization, production of reactive oxygen species (ROS), and activation of ERK1/2 MAPK and Akt pathways and increases cell proliferation in MCF-7 cells [80]. BPAF also upregulates GPER-1 and ERα protein expression whereas silencing of GPER-1 markedly reduced BPAF-stimulated cell proliferation [80]. Furthermore, 4,4′-thiodiphenol (TDP), another molecule derived from BPA, has similar effects to those produced by BPA [81]. By activating GPER-1 signaling, BPA has also been shown to increase migration and proliferation of bovine vascular endothelial cells and SKBR3 and MDA-MB-231 breast cancer cells *in vitro* and to promote tumor growth *in vivo* [82]. Furthermore, treatment of endothelial cells with BPA, but under hypoxic conditions, induced the expression of HIF-1α (hypoxia-inducible factor-1 alpha) and VEGF (vascular endothelial growth factor) [82]. These observations support the hypothesis that BPA, through the biological activity of vascular endothelial cells, promotes the development of breast tumor cells via GPER-1.

The inflammatory response is an important component of many diseases, including metabolic diseases and cancer. Notably, BPA and BPS promote persistent inflammatory states through increased expression of IL-19, EGFR, and TGF-β, among other regulatory molecules [82, 83]. Interestingly, biological fluids from cancer patients contain elevated levels of the bioactive peptide hormones known as kinins [84], and the kinin B1 receptor (B1R), another member of the GPCR family stimulated by kinin B1R agonists (Lys-des[Arg^9]bradykinin or des[Arg^9]bradykinin), is expressed in ductal breast carcinoma *in situ*, invasive ductal carcinoma, and benign fibroadenomas [84, 85]. In addition, we have previously determined that stimulation of kinin B1R promotes cell proliferation, chemotaxis, and release of metalloproteinases (MMP-2 and MMP-9) from breast cancer cells through the EGFR/ERK1/2 pathway [85, 86]. Although there is no research directly linking bisphenol activity with the kinin B1R, we have recently reported that both GPER-1 and B1R are overexpressed in ERα-positive breast cancer cells continuously exposed to tamoxifen [64], suggesting a possible cross-talk between both GPCRs in estrogen-sensitive breast cancer cells, to increase cell proliferation and cancer progression under persistent exposure to bisphenols. If other GPCRs of the GPER-1 family such as the orphan GPCR, GPR161 (G protein-coupled receptor 161), is activated by bisphenols, it is an unexplored and interesting field since GPR161 is overexpressed in TNBCs and correlates with a bad prognosis. Overexpression of GPR161 in human mammary epithelial cells produces an increase in cell proliferation, migration, intracellular accumulation of E-cadherin, formation of multiacinar structures in 3D cell cultures, and invasion through a rapamycin signaling-dependent pathway [87].

4.4 Angiotensin receptors

Specific angiotensin-binding sites in tissues were discovered in the 1960s by Merlin Bumpus, following tracking of radioactive angiotensin infused into live rats [88]. The physiological relevance of this finding was related to the best-known responses triggered by angiotensins, such as vasoconstriction or aldosterone secretion [88, 89]. Subsequently, the specific and saturable binding of radiolabeled angiotensin was demonstrated in homogenates, subcellular fractions, and tissues of several species, including humans [90]. Additionally, pharmacological experiments showed different tissue responses to angiotensin and the presence of different types of angiotensin receptor (AT) proteins [91, 92]. The classification of angiotensin receptors was initially somewhat confusing, but today two types of receptors are formally recognized and called AT1 and AT2 [93–95]. The human AT1 receptor is encoded by a single gene located on the q arm, band 22 of chromosome 3 and its distribution is quite wide in adult tissues [89, 94]. AT1 activation triggers an intracellular signaling cascade that promotes the phosphorylation of proteins that participate in smooth muscle contraction, aldosterone secretion, cell growth, and cell proliferation [96]. By comparison, the gene that encodes the AT2 receptor is located on the X chromosome [93], expressing itself predominantly during intrauterine development though its levels have been found to increase due to stress or tissue damage [96]. Physiologically, the activity of AT2 receptor antagonizes that of the AT1 receptor [94, 96]. Since their discovery, angiotensin receptors have been considered important therapeutic targets for hypertension, heart and kidney failure, and other types of vascular diseases [10]. Moreover, angiotensin receptors have also been involved in the development of different types of metabolic and neoplastic diseases.

One of the most important theories elaborated to explain the origin and persistence of cancer in modern societies deals with CSCs, key cellular players first isolated in the 1990s by John E. Dick from human acute myeloid leukemia cells [97]. So far, CSCs have been identified in different types of tumors as a subpopulation of cancer cells with self-renewal and multipotency properties, capable of initiating and maintaining carcinogenesis, through clones with different degrees of differentiation, and responsible for resistance to treatment strategies, metastases, and disease relapse [34, 98]. Recent evidence indicates that the RAS pathway is crucial for an appropriate tumor microenvironment and maintenance and differentiation of CSCs [36, 97–99].

Overexpression of the AT2 receptor stimulates the differentiation of mesenchymal stem cells [99], and signaling via AT1 or AT2 receptors can condition the hematopoietic lineage [98]. Expression of angiotensin receptors and other members of the RAS pathway in CSCs suggests that new therapeutic routes may emerge for several types of cancer [10, 100–102]. Human embryonic cells exposed to low concentrations of BPA upregulate the expression of Oct4 and Nanog proteins, two early differentiation markers of mammary epithelial cells [103]. Another possible regulator of CSCs, activated by BPA, is bone morphogenetic protein [104]; it has been suggested that bone morphogenetic protein 2 initiates the transformation of stem cells toward a malignant phenotype [105]. Similarly, the presence of angiotensin II has been verified in breast cancer epithelial cells [102, 106] and the stroma [102] and overexpression of AT1 receptor in MCF-7 cells has been associated with an increased capacity for cell migration, invasion, proliferation [101, 107], and release of MMP-9 [107], responses associated with phosphorylation of ERK1/2 MAPK [107]. Interestingly, most of the effects of angiotensin II on cell proliferation and activation of the Ras-Raf-MAPK pathway and the transcription factors NF-κB and CREB can be inhibited by an AT1 interfering RNA, plus treatment with irbesartan, an AT1 pharmacological antagonist [107]. On the other hand, a study in nonmetastatic operable breast tumors determined the presence of AT2 receptors in up to 35% of cases whereas tumors expressing the AT1 receptor corresponded to stage III and showed an increased number of mitosis and vascularization [108].

Considering that inflammation and increased angiogenesis are two events directly associated with angiotensin receptors' dysregulation, these receptors have been proposed to contribute significantly to the development of neoplasia, especially if we consider the possibility that they could be activated by bisphenols [107–109].

4.5 Chemokine receptors

Evolutionarily, it is estimated that the origin of the chemokine system dates back about 650 million years ago [110]. This system has undergone great structural and functional diversification, contributing to the physiological activity of the different tissues of vertebrates [110, 111]. The first chemokine was described in 1977 by identifying the sequence and activity of platelet factor 4 (PF-4) [112]. In 1985, gamma interferon, another chemokine with high homology with PF-4 and proinflammatory activity, was discovered [113]. Subsequently, Yoshimura et al. isolated and described a monocyte chemotactic protein (MCP-1), which is currently recognized as one of the most potent monocyte activators [114]. Initially, chemokines were given names associated with their biological activity, but in order to limit the generation of a diversity of names due to the increasing amount of chemokines discovered, a nomenclature was created in the year 2000 [115]. Currently, chemokines are characterized by the presence of four cysteine residues involved in their 3-dimensional shape; chemokines are classified into four main subfamilies: CC, CXC, XC, and CX3C followed by a number (the "X" corresponds to an amino acid that can change) [115].

At the beginning of the 1990s it was determined that stimulation of leukocytes by proinflammatory chemokines induced a transient increase in intracellular calcium levels [116, 117]; this observation constituted one of the first indications of chemokine receptors' activity such as GPCRs-dependent chemokines [111, 115]. Initially it was thought that the activity of chemokine receptors was limited to modulation of certain aspects of the immune response, such as the recruitment of neutrophils during acute inflammation or of monocytes during chronic inflammation. However, it is currently considered that practically any cell type in the body can express chemokine receptors and not just leukocytes [111, 118]. Similarly, it is estimated that around 20 chemokine receptors can recognize the more than 50 chemokines studied so far [118, 119]. This opens a range of biological responses commanded by chemokine receptors and accounts for versatility of these receptors in their interaction with chemokines including a role in the pathophysiology of cancer. The first investigation that evidenced this activity used a model of murine lymphoma and demonstrated the association between MCP-1 (current CCL2) with promotion of tissue invasion [120]. Following this finding, the activity of chemokine receptors in the initiation and progression of different types of cancers has been demonstrated [111, 121]. In breast cancer, chemokine receptors can downregulate the immune response, favoring tumor progression [119, 121] by promoting tumor growth and survival signals [119]. The chemokine system has also been related to the maintenance of CSCs, through modulation of tumor microenvironment [111, 119, 121]. Although there are still many factors to be clarified, it has been established that the chemokine system significantly strengthens carcinogenic activity by promoting angiogenesis. Actually, the chemokine receptors expressed in endothelial cells and displaying high proangiogenic activity are CXCR2 (whose ligands are CXCL1, CXCL2, CXCL3, CXCL5, CXCL6, CXCL7, and CXCL8), and CXCR1 (whose ligand is CXCL8, one of the most potent angiogenic molecules) [119]. Additionally, it is known that CXCL8 induces higher levels of MMP-2 and MMP-9 and of VEGF, supporting its role in cancer cell migration and metastasis [111]. Recently, CXCL1-3 has been negatively correlated with the prognosis and survival of breast cancer patients [122]. Furthermore, a phytoestrogen, called quercetin (a flavonoid found in high concentrations in fruits and vegetables), has been found to have an inhibitory effect on cell proliferation, promoting apoptosis in MDA-MB-231 and MCF-7 cells and increasing CXCL1-2 secretion [122].

It has been suggested that early exposure to BPA can cause deleterious immunological effects, creating over time the organic conditions for development of a variety of disorders during adulthood; thus, bisphenols can dysregulate the chemokine network altering homeostasis of the immune system. A study in which a low dose of BPA was administered intratracheally in six-week-old male mice suggests that BPA exacerbates the allergic process of the airways through the expression of CXCR4 receptors in antigen-presenting cells [123]. Additionally, it has been estimated that 10 μM BPA, BPS, and BPAF increase secretion levels of chemokines, such as CXCL8 (IL-8), reducing the viability of human macrophages [124]; this effect is partially reversed by exposure to genistein (one of the most common phytoestrogens) [124].

Notably, 17β-estradiol increases the expression of CXC12 and its receptor CXCR4 in MCF-7 cells but inhibits the expression of CXCR7, the other receptor for this chemokine. Overexpression of CXC12 and CXCR4 is important for the increase in the proliferation rate of breast cancer cells stimulated with 17β-estradiol. By contrast, high levels of CXCR7 are related to the basal growth of tumor cells [125]. These effects can be explained molecularly by the regulatory effect of 17β-estradiol on the level of chromatin compaction in the promoters of genes related to chemokines.

Furthermore, the activity of the chemokine network has been associated with a series of estrogenic compounds in estrogen-sensitive breast cancer cells. Genistein and BPA (in addition to estrogen) have been shown to stimulate CXC12 synthesis and secretion in T47D breast cancer cells [126]. Similarly, it has been observed that BPAF stimulates proliferation of T47D cells, in a dose-dependent manner, promoting transcription and secretion of CXCL12, while the use of a shRNA or selective inhibition of CXCL12 significantly reduced the activity of CXCL12 and cell proliferation [127]. Dysregulation of the chemokine network by BPs has been associated, in humans and animals, with a variety of adverse effects both on the development and on the structure of the mammary gland, highlighting the generation of intraductal hyperplasia and carcinoma *in situ* in mice exposed prenatally to BPA [128]. Thus, early exposure to BPA may increase susceptibility of the mammary gland to malignant transformation. Notably, prenatal exposure of mice to BPA induced gene reprogramming that resulted in low expression of members of the CXC family (CXCL2, CXCL4, CXCL14, and CXCL20) and of the interferon regulatory factor 9 (IL-R9) as well as the immune response gene 1 (Irg1) and some members of genes 1 (IL-1β and IL1-RN) and genes 2 (IL-7) of the interleukin family [129]. These changes affected the normal activity of the inflammatory response, increasing the risk of developing breast cancer in the long term [129].

In perspective, the set of experimental results indicates that bisphenols, particularly BPA and BPAF, target the mammary gland, affecting the expression of chemokine receptors and their ligands, alterations that have been associated with changes in normal development. Although an important part of the research indicates a possible cross-talk between nuclear estrogen receptors, GPCRs and bisphenols to alter homeostasis of the chemokine system, this interactions have so far not been directly addressed and remain largely unknown.

4.6 Adrenergic receptors

Epinephrine and norepinephrine bind to specific GPCRs referred to as adrenergic receptors, modulating physiological responses such as metabolism, vascular tone, and cell proliferation. These receptors are classified into three types, which are subdivided into the following subtypes: α1-adrenergic (α1A, α1B, α1D), α2-adrenergic (α2A, α2B, α2C), and β-adrenergic (β1, β2, β3) [130, 131]. In general, α-adrenergic receptors have a vasoconstrictive effect and produce excitation in the uterus, heart, and blood vessels and have a relaxing effect in the intestine [132]. On the other hand, β-adrenergic receptors have a vasodilator effect, but a vasoconstrictor activity in the uterus and an excitatory effect in the myocardium [131, 132]. By binding to catecholamines, AR activate various signaling pathways that depend on heterotrimeric G proteins, which use phospholipase C and adenyl cyclase to produce second messengers that activate cytosolic kinases, which by translocating to the nucleus modulate different transcription factors [133]. Two single nucleotide polymorphisms of the α2-adrenergic receptor gene (rs1800544 and rs553668) have been considered as useful tools to predict the severity of invasive breast cancer and their relation with metabolic alterations [130]. Presence of AR has been described in human epithelial breast cells [134, 135] and in adipocytes of breast tissue [131, 136]. Furthermore, stimulation of α and β AR by catecholamines has been shown to stimulate proliferation and migration of non-tumor (MCF-10A) and neoplastic (MCF-7 and MDA-MB-231) breast epithelial cells, generating an increase in cAMP levels, effects that are reversed by the use of AR antagonists [135, 136].

Prenatal exposure of mice to BPA (10 μg/kg body weight) and its binding to α2-adrenergic receptors changed the binding affinity of adrenaline to α2-adrenergic receptors in the locus coeruleus and the medial preoptic area of the brain and eliminated the behavioral differences between males and females related to emotion and anxiety [137]. Other studies have indicated that intrauterine exposure to BPA can alter the programming of most sensitive brain regions to steroids, differentially affecting men and women [51, 138]. On the other hand, both BPA and BPS have been shown to promote lipid accumulation and differentiation of murine 3 T3-L1 adipocytes in a dose-dependent manner though BPS displayed more adipogenicity than BPA [136]. Interestingly, it has been established that alterations in the typical responses of the sympathetic nervous system and its signaling pathways alter the normal metabolic balance, generating conditions for the establishment of disorders, such as obesity and type II diabetes mellitus, and consequently increasing the risk for cancer development [133].

Although there is no conclusive evidence to establish a direct relationship between bisphenols exposure and activation of AR in the context of breast cancer, experimental evidence indicates that they are involved in the development of breast cancer at a systemic level mediated by the sympathetic nervous system and through activation of α and β adrenergic receptors that are expressed in a great variety of cell types, including epithelial cells and adipocytes of the breast. On the other hand, interactions of AR with BPA in cells of the nervous system and with BPA and BPS during adipogenesis suggest that there exists a disruptor axis in sympathetic and metabolic activity to favor the development of neoplasia [136].

5. Conclusion

Although the concern about the deleterious effects of BPA on health has been recognized by the industry, in particular its relationship with cancer, the generation of new analogs such as BPB, BPF, and BPAF, which are part of products labeled as BPA-free, has not solved the problem [129]. Indeed, *in vitro* assays have revealed that BPAF has a stronger binding affinity for estrogen receptors than BPA [80]. The evidence accumulated so far suggests that BPA and BPS may contribute to breast cancer by disrupting the organization of acinar structures and by affecting the natural development of the mammary gland [3]. To date, the effects of BPA in eukaryotic cells have been reported to be mediated primarily by steroid receptors, including ERα and ERβ, but also as we discussed in this chapter, the effects are also mediated by activation of GPCRs exposed on the cell surface (**Figure 2**) [41].

More studies regarding the effects of bisphenols on angiotensin, adrenergic, chemokines, B1R, or even GPER-1 receptors are necessary to determine the real risks of these compounds for human health and the particular risk of developing cancer.

Understanding the role of endocrine disruptors and the mechanisms involved in their action is crucial to prevent the harm that bisphenols may cause in the population and to improve public health approaches to control cancer as well as some chronic diseases that afflict adult life.

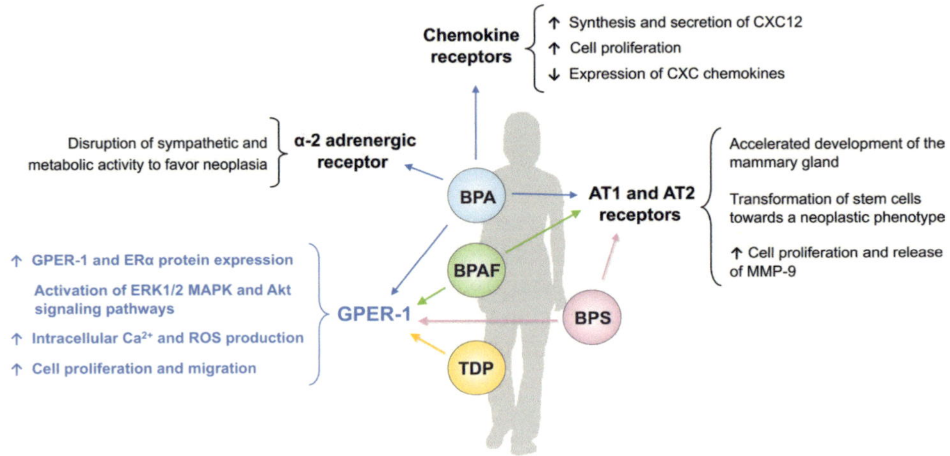

Figure 2.
Potential effects of bisphenols on GPCRs to favor development and progression of breast cancer. BPA, BPAF, BPS, bisphenols A, AF and S; GPER-1, G protein coupled estrogen receptor 1; AT, angiotensin; Erα, estrogen receptor alpha; TDP, 4,4′-thiodiphenol; ROS, reactive oxygen species.

Author details

Luis Molina[1*], Carlos D. Figueroa[2,3] and Pamela Ehrenfeld[2,3*]

1 Facultad de Medicina y Ciencia, Universidad San Sebastián, Sede De la Patagonia, Puerto Montt, Chile

2 Laboratory of Cellular Pathology, Institute of Anatomy, Histology and Pathology, Universidad Austral de Chile, Valdivia, Chile

3 Centro Interdisciplinario de Estudios del Sistema Nervioso (CISNe), Chile

*Address all correspondence to: luis.molina@uss.cl; ingridehrenfeld@uach.cl

References

[1] Dumitrascu MC, Mares C, Petca RC, Sandru F, Popescu RI, Mehedintu C, et al. Carcinogenic effects of bisphenol A in breast and ovarian cancers. Oncology Letters. 2020;**20**:282-289. DOI: 10.3892/ol.2020.12145

[2] Liao C, Kannan K. Widespread occurrence of bisphenol A in paper and paper products: Implications for human exposure. Environmental Science & Technology. 2011;**45**:9372-9379

[3] Feldman D, Krishnan A. Estrogens in unexpected places: Possible implications for researchers and consumers. Environmental Health Perspectives. 1995;**103**:129-133

[4] Hengstler JG, Foth H, Gebel T, Kramer PJ, Lilienblum W, Schweinfurth H, et al. Critical evaluation of key evidence on the human health hazards of exposure to bisphenol A. Critical Reviews in Toxicology. 2011;**41**:263-291

[5] Eladak S, Grisin T, Moison D, Guerquin MJ, N'Tumba-Byn T, Pozzi-Gaudin S, et al. A new chapter in the bisphenol a story: Bisphenol S and bisphenol F are not safe alternatives to this compound. Fertility and Sterility. 2015;**103**:11-21

[6] Cheryl S. Rosenfeld. Frontiers in Neuroendocrinology. 2017;**47**:123-133

[7] Pouzaud F, Thierry-Mieg M, Burga K, Vérines-Jouin L, Fiore K, et al. ANSES's Working Group on « Endocrine disruptors », ANSES's Expert Committee on « Chemicals covered by the REACh and CLP Regulations », Concerns related to ED-mediated effects of Bisphenol A and their regulatory consideration. Molecular and Cellular Endocrinology. 2018;**475**:92-106. DOI: 10.1016/j.mce.2018.02.002

[8] Kahn LG, Philippat C, Nakayama SF, Slama R, Trasande L. Endocrine-disrupting chemicals: Implications for human health. The Lancet Diabetes and Endocrinology. 2020;**8**:703-718

[9] Atlas E, Dimitrova V. Bisphenol S and Bisphenol A disrupt morphogenesis of MCF-12A human mammary epithelial cells. Scientific Reports. 2019;**9**:1-10. DOI: 10.1038/s41598-019-52505-x

[10] Dhanachandra Singh K, Karnik SS. Angiotensin receptors: Structure, function, signaling and clinical applications. Journal of Cellular Signaling. 2017;**01**:1-8

[11] Zincke T, Walter W. II. Ueber die Einwirkung von Brom und von Chlor auf Phenole: Substitutionsproducte, Pseudobromide und Pseudochloride. XI. Ueber die Einwirkung von Brom auf p-Oxydiphenylmethan. Justus Liebigs Annalen der Chemie. 1904;**334**:367-385

[12] Dodds. Endocrine-dirsupting chemical. Nature. 1936;**137**:996

[13] Casajuana N, Lacorte S. New methodology for the determination of phthalate esters, bisphenol A, bisphenol A diglycidyl ether, and nonylphenol in commercial whole milk samples. Journal of Agricultural and Food Chemistry. 2004;**52**:3702-3707

[14] Dodds EC, Goldberg L, Lawson W, Robinson R. Synthetic oestrogenic compounds related to stilbene and diphenylethane. Part I. Proceedings of the Royal Society B. 1939;**127**:140-167

[15] Krishnan V, Stathis P, Permuth SF, Tokes L, Feldman D. Bisphenol-A: Polycarbonate. Endocrinology. 1993;**6**:2279-2286. DOI: 10.1210/endo.132.6.8504731

[16] Pu Y, Gingrich JD, Steibel JP, Veiga-Lopez A. Sex-specific modulation of fetal adipogenesis by gestational Bisphenol A and Bisphenol S exposure. Endocrinology. 2017;**158**:3844-3858

[17] Diamanti-Kandarakis E, Bourguignon JP, Giudice LC, Hauser R, Prins GS, Soto AM, et al. Endocrine-disrupting chemicals: An Endocrine Society scientific statement. Endocrine Reviews. 2009;**30**:293-342

[18] VandeVoort CA, Gerona RR, Vom Saal FS, Tarantal AF, Hunt PA, Hillenweck A, et al. Maternal and fetal pharmacokinetics of oral radiolabeled and authentic bisphenol a in the rhesus monkey. PLoS One. 2016;**11**:1-16

[19] Mas S, Egido J, González-Parra E. The importance of bisphenol A, an uraemic toxin from exogenous sources, in haemodialysis patients. Nefrologia [Internet]. Sociedad Española de Nefrología. 2017;**37**:229-234. DOI: 10.1016/j.nefroe.2017.06.004

[20] Bousoumah R, Leso V, Iavicoli I, Huuskonen P, Viegas S, Porras SP, et al. Biomonitoring of occupational exposure to bisphenol A, bisphenol S and bisphenol F: A systematic review. Science of the Total Environment. 2021;**783**:146905. DOI: 10.1016/j.scitotenv.2021.146905

[21] Sarigiannis DA, Karakitsios SP, Handakas E, Simou K, Solomou E, Gotti A. Integrated exposure and risk characterization of bisphenol-A in Europe. Food and Chemical Toxicology. 2016;**98**:134-147. DOI: 10.1016/j.fct.2016.10.017

[22] Ullah A, Pirzada M, Jahan S, Ullah H, Shaheen G, Rehman H, et al. Bisphenol A and its analogs bisphenol B, bisphenol F, and bisphenol S: Comparative in vitro and in vivo studies on the sperms and testicular tissues of rats. Chemosphere. 2018;**209**:508-516. DOI: 10.1016/j.chemosphere.2018.06.089

[23] Le Fol V, Aït-Aïssa S, Sonavane M, Porcher JM, Balaguer P, Cravedi JP, et al. In vitro and in vivo estrogenic activity of BPA, BPF and BPS in zebrafish-specific assays. Ecotoxicology and Environmental Safety. 2017;**142**:150-156

[24] Bilancio A, Bontempo P, Di Donato M, Conte M, Giovannelli P, Altucci L, et al. Bisphenol a induces cell cycle arrest in primary and prostate cancer cells through EGFR/ERK/p53 signaling pathway activation. Oncotarget. 2017;**8**:115620-115631

[25] Rochester JR, Bolden AL. Bisphenol S and F: A systematic review and comparison of the hormonal activity of bisphenol a substitutes. Environmental Health Perspectives. 2015;**123**:643-650

[26] Matsushima A, Liu X, Okada H, Shimohigashi M, Shimohigashi Y. Bisphenol AF is a full agonist for the estrogen receptor ERα but a highly specific antagonist for ERβ. Environmental Health Perspectives. 2010;**118**:1267-1272

[27] Tharp AP, Maf MV, Hunt PA, Vandevoort CA, Sonnenschein C, Soto AM. Bisphenol A alters the development of the rhesus monkey mammary gland. Proceedings of the National Academy of Sciences of the United States of America. 2012;**19**:8190-8195. DOI: 10.1073/pnas.1120488109

[28] Wetherill YB, Akingbemi BT, Kanno J, McLachlan JA, Nadal A, Sonnenschein C, et al. In vitro molecular mechanisms of bisphenol A action. Reproductive Toxicology. 2007; **24**:178-198

[29] Fernandez SV, Huang Y, Snider KE, Zhou Y, Pogash TJ, Russo J. Expression and DNA methylation changes in human breast epithelial cells after bisphenol A exposure. International Journal of Oncology. 2012;**41**:369-377. DOI: 10.3892/ijo.2012.1444

[30] Dairkee SH, Luciani-Torres MG, Moore DH, Goodson WH. Bisphenol-A-induced inactivation of the p53 axis underlying deregulation of proliferation

kinetics, and cell death in non-malignant human breast epithelial cells. Carcinogenesis. 2013;**34**:703-712

[31] LaPensee EW, Tuttle TR, Fox SR, Ben-Jonathan N. Bisphenol A at low nanomolar doses confers chemoresistance in estrogen receptor-α-positive and -negative breast cancer cells. Environmental Health Perspectives. 2009;**117**:175-180

[32] Buteau-Lozano H, Velasco G, Cristofari M, Balaguer P, Perrot-Applanat M. Xenoestrogens modulate vascular endothelial growth factor secretion in breast cancer cells through an estrogen receptor-dependent mechanism. The Journal of Endocrinology. 2008;**196**:399-412

[33] Zhang W, Fang Y, Shi X, Zhang M, Wang X, Tan Y. Effect of bisphenol A on the EGFR-STAT3 pathway in MCF-7 breast cancer cells. Molecular Medicine Reports. 2012;**5**:41-47

[34] Lillo MA, Nichols C, Seagroves TN, Miranda-Carboni GA, Krum SA. Bisphenol A induces Sox2 in ER+ breast cancer stem-like cells. Hormones and Cancer. 2017;**8**:90

[35] O'Hayre M, Vázquez-Prado J, Kufareva I, Stawiski EW, Handel TM, Seshagiri S, et al. The emerging mutational landscape of G proteins and G-protein-coupled receptors in cancer. Nature Reviews. Cancer. 2013;**13**:412-424. Available from: https://www.nature.com/articles/nrc3521

[36] Young D, Waitches G, Birchmeier C, Fasano O, Wigler M. Isolation and characterization of a new cellular oncogene encoding a protein with multiple potential transmembrane domains. Cell. 1986;**45**:711-719. Available from: https://pubmed.ncbi.nlm.nih.gov/3708691/

[37] Acconcia F. The network of angiotensin receptors in breast cancer. Cell. 2020;**9**:1-14

[38] Maehle AH. A binding question: the evolution of the receptor concept. Endeavour. 2009;**33**:135-140. Available from:. DOI: 10.1016/j.endeavour.2009.09.001

[39] Maehle AH. "Receptive substances": John Newport Langley (1852-1925) and his path to a receptor theory of drug action. Medical History. 2004; **48**:153-174

[40] Lefkowitz RJ, Mukherjee C, Coverstone M, Caron MG. Stereospecific [3h](−)-alprenclol binding sites, e-adrenergic receptors and adenylate cyclase Robert. Biochemical and Biophysical Research Communications. 1974;**60**:703-709

[41] Caron MG, Srinivasan Y, Pitha J, Kociolek K, Lefkowitz RJ. Affinity chromatography of the β adrenergic receptor. The Journal of Biological Chemistry. 1979;**254**:2923-2927

[42] Cerione RA, Sibley DR, Codina J, Benovic JL, Winslow J, Neer EJ, et al. Reconstitution of a hormone-sensitive adenylate cyclase system. The pure β-adrenergic receptor and guanine nucleotide regulatory protein confer hormone responsiveness on the resolved catalytic unit. The Journal of Biological Chemistry. 1984;**259**:9979-9982

[43] Hanson MA, Stevens RC. Discovery of new GPCR biology: One receptor structure at a time. Structure. 2009;**17**:8-14. DOI: 10.1016/j.str.2008.12.003

[44] Palczewski K, Kumasaka T, Hori T, Behnke CA, Motoshima H, Fox BA, et al. Crystal structure of rhodopsin: A G protein-coupled receptor. Science. 2000;**289**:739-745

[45] Heifetz A, Schertler GFX, Seifert R, Tate CG, Sexton PM, Gurevich VV, et al. GPCR structure, function, drug discovery and crystallography: report from Academia-Industry International

Conference (UK Royal Society) Chicheley Hall, 1-2 September 2014. Naunyn-Schmiedeberg's Archives of Pharmacology. 2015;**388**:883-903

[46] Fredriksson R, Lagerström MC, Lundin LG, Schiöth HB. The G-protein-coupled receptors in the human genome form five main families. Phylogenetic analysis, paralogon groups, and fingerprints. Molecular Pharmacology. 2003;**63**:1256-1272

[47] Gacasan SB, Baker DL, Parrill AL. G protein-coupled receptors: The evolution of structural insight. AIMS Biophys [Internet]. American Institute of Mathematical Sciences. 2017;**4**:491-527. Available from: http://www.aimspress.com/article/doi/10.3934/biophy.2017.3.491

[48] Fredriksson R, Schiöth HB. The repertoire of G-protein-coupled receptors in fully sequenced genomes. Molecular Pharmacology. 2005; **67**:1414-1425

[49] Dunn HA, Orlandi C, Martemyanov KA. Beyond the ligand: Extracellular and transcellular G protein-coupled receptor complexes in physiology and pharmacology. Pharmacological Reviews. 2019; **71**:503-519

[50] Molina L, Figueroa CD, Bhoola KD, Ehrenfeld P. GPER-1/GPR30 a novel estrogen receptor sited in the cell membrane: Therapeutic coupling to breast cancer. Expert Opinion on Therapeutic Targets. 2017;**21**:755-766. DOI: 10.1080/14728222.2017.1350264

[51] Bustamante-Barrientos FA, Méndez-Ruette M, Ortloff A, Luz-Crawford P, Rivera FJ, Figueroa CD, et al. The impact of estrogen and estrogen-like molecules in neurogenesis and neurodegeneration: Beneficial or harmful? Frontiers in Cellular Neuroscience. 2021;**15**:1-19

[52] Durando M, Kass L, Perdomo V, Bosquiazzo VL, Luque EH, Muñoz-De-Toro M. Prenatal exposure to bisphenol A promotes angiogenesis and alters steroid-mediated responses in the mammary glands of cycling rats. The Journal of Steroid Biochemistry and Molecular Biology. 2011;**127**:35-43

[53] Tucker DK, Bouknight SH, Brar SS, Kissling GE, Fenton SE. Evaluation of prenatal exposure to bisphenol analogues on development and long-term health of the mammary gland in female mice. Environmental Health Perspectives. 2018;**126**(**8**):087003. DOI: 10.1289/EHP3189

[54] Cao LY, Ren XM, Li CH, Zhang J, Qin WP, Yang Y, et al. Bisphenol AF and Bisphenol B exert higher estrogenic effects than Bisphenol A via G Protein-coupled estrogen receptor pathway. Environmental Science & Technology. 2017;**51**:11423-11430

[55] Szego CM, Davis JS. Adenosine 3′,5′-monophosphate in rat uterus: acute elevation by estrogen. Proceedings of the National Academy of Sciences of the United States of America. 1967; **58**:1711-1718

[56] Toran-Allerand CD, Guan X, MacLusky NJ, Horvath TL, Diano S, Singh M, et al. ER-X: A novel, plasma membrane-associated, putative estrogen receptor that is regulated during development and after ischemic brain injury. The Journal of Neuroscience. 2002;**22**:8391-8401

[57] Boulware MI, Weick JP, Becklund BR, Kuo SP, Groth RD, Mermelstein PG. Estradiol activates group I and II metabotropic glutamate receptor signaling, leading to opposing influences on cAMP response element-binding protein. The Journal of Neuroscience. 2005;**25**:5066-5078

[58] Carmeci C, Thompson DA, Ring HZ, Francke U, Weigel RJ.

Identification of a gene (GPR30) with homology to the G-protein-coupled receptor superfamily associated with estrogen receptor expression in breast cancer. Genomics. 1997;**617**:-607, 17. DOI: 10.1006/geno.1997.4972

[59] Thomas P, Pang Y, Filardo EJ, Dong J. Identity of an estrogen membrane receptor coupled to a G protein in human breast cancer cells. Endocrinology. 2005;**146**:624-632

[60] Revankar CM, Cimino DF, Sklar LA, Arterburn JB, Prossnitz ER. A transmembrane intracellular estrogen receptor mediates rapid cell signaling. Science. 2005;**307**:1625-1630

[61] Prossnitz ER, Arterburn JB. International union of basic and clinical pharmacology. XCVII. G protein–coupled estrogen receptor and its pharmacologic modulators. Pharmacological Reviews. 2015; **67**:505-540

[62] Sharma G, Hu C, Staquicini DI, Brigman JL, Liu M, Mauvais-Jarvis F, et al. Preclinical efficacy of the GPER-selective agonist G-1 in mouse models of obesity and diabetes. Science Translational Medicine. 2020; **12**:eaau596. Available from: https://pubmed.ncbi.nlm.nih.gov/31996464/

[63] Revankar CM, Cimino DF, Sklar LA, Arterburn JB, Prossnitz ER. A transmembrane intracellular estrogen receptor mediates rapid cell signaling. Science. 2005;**307**: 1625-1630

[64] Molina L, Bustamante F, Ortloff A, Ramos I, Ehrenfeld P, Figueroa CD. Continuous exposure of breast cancer cells to tamoxifen upregulates GPER-1 and increases cell proliferation. Frontiers in Endocrinology. 2020; **1**:563165. Available from: https://www.frontiersin.org/article/10.3389/fendo.2020.563165/full

[65] Martensson UEA, Salehi SA, Windahl S, Gomez MF, Swärd K, Daszkiewicz-Nilsson J, et al. Deletion of the G protein-coupled receptor 30 impairs glucose tolerance, reduces bone growth, increases blood pressure, and eliminates estradiol-stimulated insulin release in female mice. Endocrinology. 2009;**150**:687-698

[66] Delbeck M, Golz S, Vonk R, Janssen W, Hucho T, Isensee J, et al. Impaired left-ventricular cardiac function in male GPR30-deficient mice. Molecular Medicine Reports. 2011;**4**:37-40

[67] Notas G, Kampa M, Castanas E. G protein-coupled estrogen receptor in immune cells and its role in immune-related diseases. Frontiers in Endocrinology. 2020;**11**:1-9

[68] Feldman RD, Limbird LE. GPER (GPR30): A nongenomic receptor (GPCR) for steroid hormones with implications for cardiovascular disease and cancer. Annual Review of Pharmacology and Toxicology. 2017;**57**:567-584

[69] Ignatov A, Ignatov T, Weienborn C, Eggemann H, Bischoff J, Semczuk A, et al. G-protein-coupled estrogen receptor GPR30 and tamoxifen resistance in breast cancer. Breast Cancer Research and Treatment. 2011;**128**:457-466

[70] Ignatov T, Claus M, Nass N, Haybaeck J, Seifert B, Kalinski T, et al. G-protein-coupled estrogen receptor GPER-1 expression in hormone receptor-positive breast cancer is associated with poor benefit of tamoxifen. Breast Cancer Research and Treatment. 2019;**174**:121-127. DOI: 10.1007/s10549-018-5064-8

[71] Zhou X, Lei Q, Guan K, Zhou X, Wang S, Wang Z, et al. Estrogen regulates Hippo signaling via GPER in breast cancer. The Journal of Clinical Investigation. 2015;**125**:2123-2135

[72] Piccolo S, Dupont S, Cordenonsi M. The biology of YAP/TAZ: Hippo signaling and beyond. Physiological Reviews. 2014;**94**:1287-1312

[73] Chan YT, Lai ACY, Lin RJ, Wang YH, Wang YT, Chang WW, et al. GPER-induced signaling is essential for the survival of breast cancer stem cells. International Journal of Cancer. 2020; **146**:1674-1685

[74] Luo H, Yang G, Yu T, Luo S, Wu C, Sun Y, et al. GPER-mediated proliferation and estradiol production in breast cancer-associated fibroblasts. Endocrine-Related Cancer. 2014; **21**:355-369

[75] Thomas P, Dong J. Binding and activation of the seven-transmembrane estrogen receptor GPR30 by environmental estrogens: A potential novel mechanism of endocrine disruption. The Journal of Steroid Biochemistry and Molecular Biology. 2006;**102**:175-179

[76] Ge LC, Chen ZJ, Liu HY, Zhang KS, Liu H, Huang HB, et al. Involvement of activating ERK1/2 through G protein coupled receptor 30 and estrogen receptor α/β in low doses of bisphenol A promoting growth of Sertoli TM4 cells. Toxicology Letters. 2014;**226**:81-89. DOI: 10.1016/j.toxlet.2014.01.035

[77] Pouzaud F, Thierry-Mieg M, Burga K, Vérines-Jouin L, Fiore K, Beausoleil C, et al. Concerns related to ED-mediated effects of Bisphenol A and their regulatory consideration. Molecular and Cellular Endocrinology. 2018;**475**:92-106

[78] Sheng Z, Wang C, Ren F, Liu Y, Zhu B. Molecular mechanism of endocrine-disruptive effects induced by Bisphenol A: The role of transmembrane G-protein estrogen receptor 1 and integrin α v β 3. Journal of Environmental Sciences. 2018;**75**:1-13. DOI: 10.1016/j.jes.2018.05.002

[79] Deng Q, Jiang G, Wu Y, Li J, Liang W, Chen L, et al. GPER / Hippo-YAP signal is involved in Bisphenol S induced migration of triple negative breast cancer (TNBC) cells. Journal of Hazardous Materials. 2018;**355**:1-9. DOI: 10.1016/j.jhazmat.2018.05.013

[80] Lei B, Sun S, Zhang X, Feng C, Xu J, Wen Y, et al. Bisphenol AF exerts estrogenic activity in MCF-7 cells through activation of Erk and PI3K/Akt signals via GPER signaling pathway. Chemosphere. 2019;**220**:362-370. DOI: 10.1016/j.chemosphere.2018.12.122

[81] Lei B, Peng W, Xu G, Wu M, Wen Y, Xu J, et al. Activation of G protein-coupled receptor 30 by thiodiphenol promotes proliferation of estrogen receptor α-positive breast cancer cells. Chemosphere. 2017;**169**:204-211. DOI: 10.1016/j.chemosphere.2016.11.066

[82] Xu F, Wang X, Wu N, He S, Yi W, Xiang S, et al. Bisphenol A induces proliferative effects on both breast cancer cells and vascular endothelial cells through a shared GPER-dependent pathway in hypoxia. Environmental Pollution. 2017;**231**:1609-1620. DOI: 10.1016/j.envpol.2017.09.069

[83] Segovia-Mendoza M, Gómez de León CT, García-Becerra R, Ambrosio J, Nava-Castro KE, Morales-Montor J. The chemical environmental pollutants BPA and BPS induce alterations of the proteomic profile of different phenotypes of human breast cancer cells: A proposed interactome. Environmental Research. 2020;**191**:109960-109972. DOI: 10.1016/j.envres.2020.109960

[84] Figueroa CD, Ehrenfeld P, Bhoola KD. Kinin receptors as targets for cancer therapy. Expert Opinion on Therapeutic Targets. 2012;**16**:299-312

[85] Molina L, Matus CE, Astroza A, Pavicic F, Tapia E, Toledo C, et al. Stimulation of the bradykinin B1

receptor induces the proliferation of estrogen-sensitive breast cancer cells and activates the ERK1/2 signaling pathway. Breast Cancer Research and Treatment. 2009;**118**:499-510

[86] Ehrenfeld P, Conejeros I, Pavicic MF, Matus CE, Gonzalez CB, Quest AFG, et al. Activation of kinin B1 receptor increases the release of metalloproteases-2 and -9 from both estrogen-sensitive and -insensitive breast cancer cells. Cancer Letters. 2011;**301**:106-118. DOI: 10.1016/j.canlet.2010.09.020

[87] Feigin ME, Xue B, Hammell MC, Muthuswamy SK. G-protein-coupled receptor GPR161 is overexpressed in breast cancer and is a promoter of cell proliferation and invasion. Proceedings of the National Academy of Sciences of the United States of America. 2014;**111**:4191-4196

[88] Bumpus FM, Smeby RR, Page IH, Khairallah PA. Distribution and metabolic fate of angiotensin II and various derivatives. Canadian Medical Association Journal. 1964;**90**:190-193

[89] Cherne PN, Young P. Historia del sistema renina angiotensina: Grandes hombres, un gran descubrimiento. Revista Médica de Chile. 2014; **142**:1210-1216

[90] Lin SYGT. Angiotensin receptors. The American Journal of Physiology. 1970;**218**:1319-1328

[91] Peach MJ. Renin-angiotensin system: Biochemistry and mechanisms of action. Physiological Reviews. 1977;**57**:313-370

[92] Marie-Aude D, Meyer P. Commentary angiotensin receptors. Biochemical Pharmacology. 1978;**27**:1-5

[93] Dasgupta C, Zhang. Angiotensin II receptors and drug discovery in cardiovascular disease. Drug Discovery Today. 2011;**16**:22-34. Available from: https://pubmed.ncbi.nlm.nih.gov/21147255/

[94] de Gasparo M, Catt KJ, Inagami T, Wright JWUT. International union of pharmacology. XIII. Pharmacological Reviews. 2000;**52**:415-472

[95] Allen AM, Zhuo J, Mendelsohn FAO. Localization and function of angiotensin AT1 receptors. American Journal of Hypertension. 2000;**13**:31-38

[96] Carey RM. Update on angiotensin AT2 receptors. Current Opinion in Nephrology and Hypertension. 2017;**26**:91-96

[97] Dick JE. Normal and leukemic human stem cells assayed in SCID mice. Seminars in Immunology. 1996; **8**:197-206

[98] Hubert C, Savary K, Gasc J, Corvol P. The hematopoietic system : a new niche for the renin-angiotensin system. Review Criteria in Humans. 2006;**3**:80-85

[99] Matsushita K, Wu Y, Okamoto Y, Pratt RE, Dzau VJ. Local renin angiotensin expression regulates human mesenchymal stem cell differentiation to adipocytes. Hypertension. 2006; **48**:1095-1102

[100] Roth IM, Wickremesekera AC, Wickremesekera SK, Davis PF, Tan ST. Therapeutic targeting of cancer stem cells via modulation of the renin-angiotensin system. Frontiers in Oncology. 2019;**9**:1-12

[101] Du N, Feng J, Hu L, Sun XIN, Sun H, Zhao Y, et al. Angiotensin II receptor type 1 blockers suppress the cell proliferation effects of angiotensin II in breast cancer cells by inhibiting AT1R signaling. Oncology Reports. 2012;**27**:1893-1903

[102] Vinson GP, Barker S, Puddefoot JR. The renin-angiotensin system in the

breast and breast cancer. Endocrine-Related Cancer. 2012;**19**:1-19

[103] Yang L, Luo L, Ji W, Gong C, Wu D, Huang H, et al. Effect of low dose bisphenol A on the early differentiation of human embryonic stem cells into mammary epithelial cells. Toxicology Letters. 2013;**218**:187-193. DOI: 10.1016/j.toxlet.2013.01.026

[104] Chapellier M, Maguer-Satta V. BMP2, a key to uncover luminal breast cancer origin linked to pollutant effects on epithelial stem cells niche. Molecular & Cellular Oncology. 2016;**3**:3-5

[105] Winz C, Suh N. Understanding the mechanistic link between bisphenol A and cancer stem cells: A cancer prevention perspective. Journal of Cancer Prevention. 2021;**26**:18-24

[106] Kilmister EJ, Tan ST. The role of the renin–angiotensin system in the cancer stem cell niche. Journal of Histochemistry and Cytochemistry. 2021;**24**:221554211026295-221554211026308. DOI: 10.1369/00221554211026295

[107] Oh E, Kim JY, Cho Y, An H, Lee N, Jo H, et al. Overexpression of angiotensin II type 1 receptor in breast cancer cells induces epithelial-mesenchymal transition and promotes tumor growth and angiogenesis. Biochimica et Biophysica Acta. 2016;**1863**:1071-1081. DOI: 10.1016/j.bbamcr.2016.03.010

[108] Arrieta O, Villarreal-Garza C, Vizcaíno G, Pineda B, Hernández-Pedro N, Guevara-Salazar P, et al. Association between AT1 and AT2 angiotensin II receptor expression with cell proliferation and angiogenesis in operable breast cancer. Tumor Biology. 2015;**36**:5627-5634

[109] Smith GR, Missailidis S. Cancer, inflammation and the AT1 and AT2 receptors. Journal of Inflammation. 2004;**1**:1-12

[110] DeVries ME, Kelvin AA, Xu L, Ran L, Robinson J, Kelvin DJ. Defining the origins and evolution of the chemokine/chemokine receptor system. Journal of Immunology. 2006; **176**:401-415

[111] Chen K, Bao Z, Tang P, Gong W, Yoshimura T, Wang JM. Chemokines in homeostasis and diseases. Cellular & Molecular Immunology. 2018;**15**:324-334

[112] Deuel TF, Keim PS, Farmer M, Heinrikson RL. Amino acid sequence of human platelet factor 4. Proceedings of the National Academy of Sciences of the United States of America. 1977; **74**:2256-2258

[113] Luster AD, Unkeless JC, Ravetch JV. γ-Interferon transcriptionally regulates an early-response gene containing homology to platelet proteins. Nature. 1985;**315**:672-676

[114] Yoshimura T, Matsushima K, Tanaka S, Robinson EA, Appella E, Oppenheim JJ, et al. Purification of a human monocyte-derived neutrophil chemotactic factor that has peptide sequence similarity to other host defense cytokines. Proceedings of the National Academy of Sciences of the United States of America. 1987;**84**:9233-9237

[115] Zlotnik A, Yoshie O. Chemokines: A new classification system and their role in immunity. Journal of Cultural Heritage. 2000;**1**:121-127

[116] Holmes WE, Lee J, Kuang WJ, Rice GC, Wood WI. Structure and functional expression of a human interleukin-8 receptor. Science. 1991;**253**:1278-1280

[117] Neote K, DiGregorio D, Mak JY, Horuk R, Schall TJ. Molecular cloning, functional expression, and signaling characteristics of a C-C chemokine receptor. Cell. 1993;**72**:415-425

[118] Monteagudo C, Pellín-Carcelén A, Martín JM, Ramos D. Papel de las

quimiocinas en la progresión del melanoma. Actas Dermo-Sifiliográficas. 2011;**102**:498-504

[119] King J, Mir H, Singh S. Association of cytokines and chemokines in pathogenesis of breast cancer. Progress in Molecular Biology and Translational Science. 2017;**151**:113-136. DOI: 10.1016/bs.pmbts.2017.07.003

[120] Wang JM, Chertov O, Proost P, Li JJ, Menton P, Xu L, et al. Purification and identification of chemokines potentially involved in kidney-specific metastasis by a murine lymphoma variant: Induction of migration and NFκB activation. International Journal of Cancer. 1998;**75**:900-907

[121] Korbecki J, Grochans S, Gutowska I, Barczak K, Baranowska-Bosiacka I. Cc chemokines in a tumor: A review of pro-cancer and anti-cancer properties of receptors ccr5, ccr6, ccr7, ccr8, ccr9, and ccr10 ligands. International Journal of Molecular Sciences. 2020;**21**:1-34

[122] Wang F, Yuan C, Wu HZ, Liu B, Yang YF. Bioinformatics, molecular docking and experiments in vitro analyze the prognostic value of CXC chemokines in breast cancer. Frontiers in Oncology. 2021;**11**:1-17

[123] Koike E, Yanagisawa R, Win-Shwe TT, Takano H. Exposure to low-dose bisphenol A during the juvenile period of development disrupts the immune system and aggravates allergic airway inflammation in mice. International Journal of Immunopathology and Pharmacology. 2018;**32**:2058738418774897. DOI: 10.1177/2058738418774897

[124] Chen Y, Xu HS, Guo TL. Modulation of cytokine/chemokine production in human macrophages by bisphenol a: A comparison to analogues and interactions with genistein. Journal of Immunotoxicology. 2018;**15**:96-103. DOI: 10.1080/1547691X.2018.1476629

[125] Boudot A, Kerdivel G, Habauzit D, Eeckhoute J, Le Dily F, Flouriot G, et al. Differential estrogen-regulation of CXCL12 chemokine receptors, CXCR4 and CXCR7, contributes to the growth effect of estrogens in breast cancer cells. PLoS One. 2011;**6**:2-13

[126] Habauzit D, Boudot A, Kerdivel G, Flouriot G. Development and validation of a test for environmental estrogens: Checking xeno-estrogen activity by CXCL12 secretion in breast cancer cell lines. Environmental Toxicology. 2010;**25**:495-503 Available from: https://pubmed.ncbi.nlm.nih.gov/20549624/

[127] Li M, Han X, Gao W, Chen F, Shao B. Bisphenol AF stimulates transcription and secretion of C-X-C chemokine ligand 12 to promote proliferation of cultured T47D breast cancer cells. Toxicology. 2015;**338**:30-36. DOI: 10.1016/j.tox.2015.09.007

[128] Murray TJ, Maffini MV, Ucci AA, Sonnenschein C, Soto AM. Induction of mammary gland ductal hyperplasias and carcinoma in situ following fetal bisphenol A exposure. Reproductive Toxicology. 2007;**23**:383-390. DOI: 10.1016/j.reprotox.2006.10.002

[129] Fischer C, Mamillapalli R, Goetz LG, Jorgenson E, Ilagan Y, Taylor HS. Bisphenol A (BPA) exposure in utero leads to immunoregulatory cytokine dysregulation in the mouse mammary gland: A potential mechanism programming breast cancer risk. Hormones and Cancer. 2016; 7:241-251

[130] Kaabi B, Belaaloui G, Benbrahim W, Hamizi K, Sadelaoud M, Toumi W, et al. ADRA2A germline gene polymorphism is associated to the severity, but not to the risk, of breast cancer. Pathology Oncology Research. 2016;**22**:357-365

[131] Collins S, Surwit RS. The β-adrenergic receptors and the control

of adipose tissue metabolism and thermogenesis. Recent Progress in Hormone Research. 2001;**56**:309-328

[132] Ahlquist RP. A study of the adrenotropic receptors. The American Journal of Physiology. 1948;**153**:586-600. DOI: 10.1152/ajplegacy.1948.153.3.586

[133] Dieterich LC, Bikfalvi A. The tumor organismal environment: Role in tumor development and cancer immunotherapy. Seminars in Cancer Biology. 2020;**65**:197-206. DOI: 10.1016/j.semcancer.2019.12.021

[134] Vázquez SM, Mladovan AG, Pérez C, Bruzzone A, Baldi A, Lüthy IA. Human breast cell lines exhibit functional α2-adrenoceptors. Cancer Chemotherapy and Pharmacology. 2006;**58**:50-61

[135] Amaro F, Silva D, Reguengo H, Oliveira JC, Quintas C, Vale N, et al. Β-Adrenoceptor activation in breast Mcf-10a cells induces a pattern of catecholamine production similar to that of tumorigenic Mcf-7 cells. International Journal of Molecular Sciences. 2020;**21**:1-16

[136] Ahmed S, Atlas E. Bisphenol S- and bisphenol A-induced adipogenesis of murine preadipocytes occurs through direct peroxisome proliferator-activated receptor gamma activation. International Journal of Obesity. 2016;**40**:1566-1573

[137] Ponzi D, Gioiosa L, Parmigiani S, Palanza P. Effects of prenatal exposure to a low-dose of bisphenol a on sex differences in emotional behavior and central alpha2-adrenergic receptor binding. International Journal of Molecular Sciences. 2020;**21**:3269-3283. DOI: 10.3390/ijms21093269

[138] Palanza P, Nagel SC, Parmigiani S, vom Saal FS. Perinatal exposure to endocrine disruptors: Sex, timing and behavioral endpoints. Current Opinion in Behavioral Sciences. 2016;**7**:69-75. DOI: 10.1016/j.cobeha.2015.11.017

Section 2

Pathological Conditions Related to Bisphenols

Chapter 3

The Effects of Bisphenols on Semen Quality

Parichehr Nouri and Ali Olfati

Abstract

Both the animals and humans with generalized lipodystrophy develop signs of infertility syndrome in the absence of semen health. Infertility is defined as not being able to get pregnant (conceive) after one year (or longer) of unprotected sex. The treatment of disease is usually expensive. Their expertise and experience provide the most current knowledge to promote future research. Dietary habits need to be altered, for most of world people. Therefore, the conclusions and recommendations from the part of this chapters will provide a basis for change. We welcome your offers and criticisms for book improvement in next editions. Bisphenol has been used since the 1950s, in food packaging, industrial materials, dental sealants, and personal hygiene products. Everyone is exposed to Bisphenol through the skin, inhalation, and digestive system. Bisphenol disrupts endocrine pathways because it has weak estrogenic, antiandrogenic, and antithyroid activities. Known endocrine disruptor bisphenol A (BPA) has been shown to be a reproductive toxicant in animal models. This book chapter the current epidemiological literature on fertility outcomes associated with Bisphenol exposure. It also provides relevant resources for health care providers who are in a unique position to provide guidance in reducing exposure to this endocrine-disrupting chemical.

Keywords: Semen, Bishphenol A, Infertility, Regenerative medicine

1. Introduction

Semen is the result of secretions from different parts of the ducts and glands, so that the secretions Ferrous seminiferous tubules 5%, seminal vesicle secretions 70%, and prostate secretions 25% make it [1].

Semen is examined macroscopically and microscopically:

a. Macroscopic features include:

1. Appearance: Semen has a whitish gray appearance. Red or brown color indicates blood in the semen, and yellow color indicates some vitamins, drugs or hepatitis, and indicates abnormality.

2. Liquefaction: Liquidation is a natural process in the consistency of semen that changes from a semi-liquid to a liquid state.

3. Viscosity: The viscosity can be checked by inserting a glass rod into the sample and observing its elongation after gently removing the rod.

4. Volume: The volume of human semen is at least 1.5 ml, which is measured through a graduated pipette with a sensitivity of 0.1 ml. The volume of semen is mainly due to the secretions of the prostate glands and seminal vesicles and a small amount is due to the secretions of the bulbo urethral glands and the epididymes.

5. PH: The acidity of semen reflects the balance between the acidity of different secretions of the gonads. The agreed threshold for minimum semen acidity is 7.2.

b. Microscopic features include:

1. Aggregation: Attachment of immobile sperm to each other or to mucosal masses, non-sperm cells or cell debris, as Non-specific adhesion is considered.

2. Agglutination: Refers to the attachment of motile sperm to the head to head, tail to tail, or other states they are stuck together.

3. Motility: Number of repetitions usually Depending on the volume of semen, it is defined between 2 to 3 times.

4. Vitality: In general, the percentage of live sperm is higher than motile sperm. Minimum sperm viability (health of sperm membrane) (58%) Is obtained by multiplying the total number of sperm in the percentage of healthy sperm.

5. Concentration: The number of sperm in the semen is calculated using the sperm concentration. Sperm concentration refers to the number of sperm per unit volume of semen.

2. Semen quality health

There is ample evidence in the world that global sperm quality has declined over the past few decades [2]. The probable cause of global decreased semen quality may be environmental and / or occupational and lifestyle factors [3, 4]. Lifestyle factors associated with male infertility include: smoking, alcohol consumption, recreational drugs, stress, obesity, paternal age, diet, and coffee consumption. Other factors include: testicular heat stress, cycling, lack of sleep, and cell phone magnetic waves [5].

2.1 Smoking

Research has reported that sperm concentrations in men who smoke are 17–13% lower than in men who do not smoke [6]. In addition, smoking has a negative relationship with sperm motility, sperm morphology and sperm count. Decreased semen quality is more common in men who smoke more than 20 cigarettes a day, or on average 10–20 cigarettes a day, than in men who smoke 1–10 cigarettes a day. The effect size is larger in infertile men than in the general population [7]. In addition to the detrimental effect on male fertility, smoking is responsible for DNA damage, aneuploidy and mutations in sperm [8].

2.2 Alcohol

A meta-analysis of 16,395 men showed that alcohol consumption had a detrimental effect on sperm morphology and semen volume [9]. Alcohol canimpair the process of production and maturation and morphological development of spermatozoa [10]. Spermatogenesis appears to decrease with increasing alcohol consumption [11]. Complete or partial cessation of spermatogenesis and Sertoli cell-only syndrome is much more common among heavy drinkers than non-drinkers [12].

2.3 Recreational drugs

opiates (narcotics), methamphetamines, anabolic–androgenic steroids, Marijuana, and cocaine are examples of illicit drugs thatNegatively affects male fertility. Destructive effects of these drugs is on the hypothalamic–pituitary-gonadal axis, testicular structure and sperm function [13].

2.4 Obesity

Overweight and obesity cause excessive accumulation of fat in the body, which is determined by using the body mass index. Men who are overweight and obese are more likely to have low sperm quality and infertility. A systematic review of 30 studies involving 158,115 men found that paternal obesity was associated with reduced male fertility. Obese men have a higher percentage of sperm with fragmented DNA, mitochondria with low membrane potential, abnormal morphology, and infertility [14].

2.5 Psychological stress

Stress, in all its forms, is detrimental to male reproductive potential. The classical stress response activates the sympathetic nervous system and engages the cytothalamic-pituitary–adrenal (HPA) axis [15]. The HPA axis and gonadotrophin-inhibitory hormone (GnIH) have an inhibitory effect on testicular Leydig cells and the hypothalamic–pituitary-gonadal axis. This inhibitory effect reduces testosterone levels. This causes changes in the Sertoli cells and the blood-testicular barrier, which eventuallysuppress spermatogenesis [16].

2.6 Advanced paternal age

There is no clear definition ofAdvanced paternal age. Studies have defined this age as between 35 and 50 years with a classification in the age range of 5 years [17]. A meta-analysis of 90 studies involving 93839 participants stated that sperm volume, total sperm count, normal sperm morphology, and progressive sperm motility decreased with age and sperm DNA fragmentation increased with age. However, sperm concentration was not significantly associated with increasing age of men [18].

2.7 Diet

Nutrition and diet have a great impact on sperm quality. Balanced and proper nutrition improves fertility and sperm quality [19]. High-fat dairy, coffee, alcohol, sugary drinks, and processed meats are associated with low sperm quality and low fertility. Low-fat dairy products, grains, poultry and fish, vegetables and fruits increase sperm quality [19].

2.8 Other lifestyle risk factor

An important risk factor for male infertility is genital heat stress caused by increased scrotal temperature. Varicocele, exposure to radiant heat, cryptorchidism, and prolonged sitting can all lead to testicular heat stress [20]. Increased scrotal temperature leads to spermatogenicsuppression, sperm DNA damage, oxidative stress andgerm cell apoptosis [21]. Cycling is associated with an increase in testicular temperature [22]. The detrimental effects of sleep disorders on male fertility are likely, as semen volume is lower in patients who have difficulty starting to sleep, such as smokers and alcoholics [23]. Radio frequencies emitted from a mobile phone and exposed to magnetic radiation can have devastating effects on the testicles [24]. A study has shown that exposure to mobile radiation can reduce sperm motility and viability [25], While another study showed that these destructive effects occur only in vitro [26].

The role of environmental pollution is critical because of its impact on sperm quality [27]. Since 1960, the rate of male infertility in industrialized countries has risen from 7–35% [28]. Research has shown with certainty that environmental toxins have a detrimental effect on male fertility in many ways. These toxins reduce the number and function of sperm [29]. The worst toxins that interfere with fertility bisphenol A (BPA), organochlorine compounds (chlorinated pesticides, polychlorinated biphenyls, and dioxins), and organophosphate pesticides and herbicides. However, many other chemicals, metals, and air pollutants seriously damage fertility [29]. In infertile couples, mercury levels were significantly higher than in the control group [30]. There is a significant relationship between blood cadmium levels in men and infertility [31].

3. Bisphnol A

The plastic monomer and plasticizer BPA is one of the chemicals produced worldwide, producing more than 66 million pound a year [32]. BPA is used in the production of epoxy resins and polycarbonate plastics used in metal cans and in many plastic products, including water pipes, sports safety equipment, dental monomers, toys, spectacle lenses and pipes [33]. Oral exposure to bisphenol A occurs more frequently. Another possible route that exposes humans to bisphenols is by inhalation and through the skin [34].

3.1 Metabolism and toxicokinetics

Bisphenol is metabolized in the liver by uridine 5-disphospho-glucuronyl transferase (UGT), and is catalyzed by glucuronidation (**Figure 1**) [35].

BPA interacts with estrogen receptors due to its phenolic structure and acts as an antagonist and agonist through endocrine receptor-dependent (ER) signaling pathways [36]. Accordingly, BPA appears to play a role in the pathogenesis of endocrine disorders including infertility in both men and women [37].

As the concentration of BPA in the urine increases, the number of sperm per ejaculation decreases. It also reduces sperm motility and sperm viability [38]. The results of clinical research conducted in recent decades have shown that the destructive effects on the endocrine glands of bisphenol A on male reproductive function, possible mechanisms by which bisphenol A may regulate spermatogenesis, mainly through the hypothalamic–pituitary-gonadal axis Specify to be involved [39]. In rodent models, with the exception of some cases, in vitro exposure to BPA at different doses (largely ranging from2 μg/kg/day to 960 mg BPA/kg body

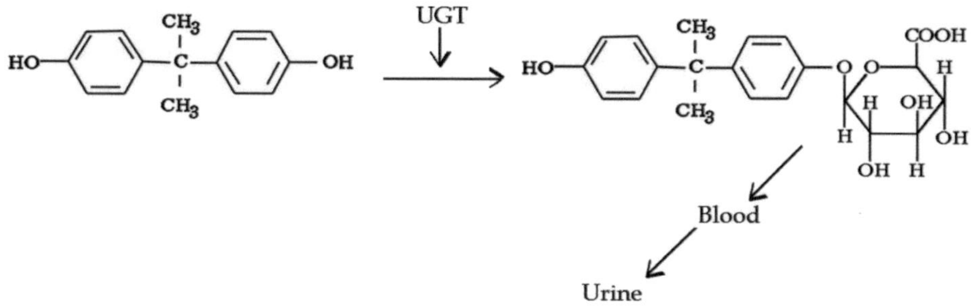

Figure 1.
Structure of bisphenol.

weight/day) and time intervals (from 5 to 84 days) caused a significant reduction in sperm count [40–43], sperm motility [41, 44], normal sperm morphology [42], increase in sperm DNA damage [44], and poor spermatogenesis [45, 46]. In a study adjusted using linear regression of confounders, increased urinary BPA levels were significantly associated with decreased total sperm count, decreased sperm motility, decreased sperm viability, and decreased sperm concentration [47]. BPA can affect sperm density and quality [48].

3.2 Resource review

1. Hatch pollard et al. reported that Higher exposure to BPA was associated with abnormal sperm tail morphology in their prospective, pre-conception cohort [49].

2. Ghada ali omran et al. reported that Total BPA levels were negatively associated with semen quality and antioxidant levels, and positively correlated with DNA damage, especially with multiple semen profile defects, alongside seminal-plasma lipid peroxidation [50].

3. Evdochia Adoamnei et al. showed that BPA exposure may be associated with a reduction in Leydig cell capacity (increased LH levels) and decreased sperm counts in young men [51].

4. Honglei Ji et al. reported that environmental exposure to BPA in a less industrialized area of China, where human urine BPA level is relatively lower, is associated with decreased sperm concentration. Impaired spermatogenesis and sperm movement may explain male subfertility resulting from exposure to BPA, although the biological mechanism is still uncertain and, therefore, needs to be disclosed by future studies [52].

5. Juan li et al. in their study showed that the, testis coefficient, sperm density, sperm activity, sperm survival rate decreased, but the sperm abnormality rate increased with increasing BPA concentrations [53].

6. Chigrinets S.V. et al. showed in their study that BPA in the seminal fluid influences negatively on the quality of the sperm and suppress the level of total testosterone in plasma [54].

7. Knez j et al. found that increased urinary BPA concentrations (5th–95th percentiles 0.3–6.7) ng/mL) were associated with lower sperm count, sperm concentration, and sperm vitality [55].

8. D.pan et al. findings identified that bisphenol A exposure may negatively contribute to the sperm quality in adult mice. Mechanistically, we showed that bisphenol A reduced sperm chromatin integrity along with increased DNA damage, which may be due to poor protamination of spermatozoa [56].

9. Ramy abou ghayda et al. found associations of urinary BPS concentrations with lower ejaculate volume, sperm concentration, total count and motility [57].

10. Alexandra E. Goldstone et al. showed A negative relation between Bisphenol and DNA fragmentation in sole significant finding in adjusted linear regression ($\beta = -0.0544$, $p = 0.035$) and suggestive of less sperm DNA damage [58].

4. Conclusions

In sum, BPA associated to male infertility. Future research will need to expand on these findings to provide a clearer picture of the effects BPAs may have on ovarian development and function, the authors wrote.

Funding

None declared.

Competing interests

None.

Authors' contributions

All authors have accepted responsibility for the entire content of this book chapter and approved its submission.

Author details

Parichehr Nouri[1] and Ali Olfati[2]*

1 Departmentof Midwifery, School of Nursing and Midwifery, Kermanshah University of Medical Sciences, Kermanshah, Iran

2 Young Researchers and Elites Club, Kermanshah Branch, Islamic Azad University, Kermanshah, Iran

*Address all correspondence to: aliolfati66@yahoo.com

References

[1] Organization SWH. WHO laboratory manual for the Examination and processing of human semen. fifth edition ed. ; 2010.

[2] Sengupta P, Borges Jr E, Dutta S, Krajewska-Kulak E. Decline in sperm count in European men during the past 50 years. Human & Experimental Toxicology. 2018;37(3):247-55.

[3] Jurewicz J RM, Sobala W, Radwan P, Bochenek M,, W. H. Effects of occupational exposure - is there a link between exposure based on an occupational questionnaire and semen quality? Syst Biol Reprod Med. 2014;60:27-32.

[4] Sharma R BK, Fedor JM, Agarwal A. Lifestyle factors and reproductive health: taking control of your fertility. Reprod Biol Endocrinol. 2013;7827-11-66.

[5] Durairajanayagam D. Lifestyle causes of male infertility. Arab Journal of Urology. 2018;16:101-20.

[6] Vine MF MB, Morrison HI, Hulka BS. Cigarette smoking and sperm density: a meta-analysis. Fertil Steril. 1994;61:35-43.

[7] Sharma R HA, Agarwal A, Esteves SC. Cigarette smoking and semen quality: a new meta-analysis examining the effect of the 2010 world health organization laboratory methods for the examination of human semen. Eur Urol. 2016;70:635-45.

[8] Beal MA, Yauk CL, Marchetti F. From sperm to offspring: Assessing the heritable genetic consequences of paternal smoking and potential public health impacts. Mutation research/ Reviews in mutation research. 2017;773:26-50.

[9] Ricci E, Al Beitawi S, Cipriani S, Candiani M, Chiaffarino F, Viganò P, et al. Semen quality and alcohol intake: a systematic review and meta-analysis. Reproductive biomedicine online. 2017;34(1):38-47.

[10] Emanuele MA EN. Alcohol's effects on male reproduction. Alcohol Health Res World. 1998; ;22:195-201.

[11] Pajarinen J KP, Savolainen V, Lalu K, Penttila A,, P. L. Moderate alcohol consumption and disorders of human spermatogenesis. Alcohol Clin Exp Res. 1996.;;20:332-7.

[12] Pajarinen JT KP. . Spermatogenic arrest and 'Sertoli cell-only' syndrome–common alcohol-induced disorders of the human testis. . Int J Androl. 1994;;17:292-9

[13] Fronczak CM KE, Barqawi AB The insults of illicit drug use on male fertility. J Androl. . 2012;;33:515-28.

[14] Campbell JM LM, Owens JA, Bakos HW. Paternal obesit negatively affects male fertility and assisted reproduction outcomes: a systematic review and meta-analysis. Reprod Biomed Online. 2015;;31:593-604.

[15] AV. M. Effects of psychological stress on male reproduction: a review. Arch Androl 1984;;13:1-7.

[16] VH. N. Effects of psychological stress on male fertility. Nat Rev Urol. 2015;;12:373-82.

[17] Wu C LL, Kovac JR. The role ofadvanced paternal age in modern reproductive medicine. Asian. J Androl. 2016;18:425.

[18] Johnson SL DJ, Gemmell NJ, Nakagawa S. . Consistent age-dependent declines in human semen quality: a systematic review and meta-analysis. Ageing Res Rev. 2015;19: 22-33.

[19] Salas-Huetos A BM, Salas-Salvado J. Dietary patterns, foods and nutrients in male fertility parameters and fecundability: a systematic review of observational studies. Hum Reprod Update. 2017;23:371-89.

[20] Durairajanayagam D SR, Du Plessis SS, Agarwal A. Testicular heat stress and sperm quality. In: Du Plessis SS, editor Male infertility: a complete guide to lifestyle and environmental factors New York: Springer Science+Business Media. 2014.

[21] Durairajanayagam D AA, Ong C. Causes,. effects and molecular mechanisms of testicular heat stress. Reprod Biomed Online. 2015;30:14-27.

[22] Maleki BH TB, Vaamonde D. . The effects of 16 weeks of intensive cycling training on seminal oxidants and antioxidants in male road cyclists. Clin J Sport Med 2014; 7: 33-41.

[23] Viganò P, Chiaffarino F, Bonzi V, Salonia A, Ricci E, Papaleo E, et al. Sleep disturbances and semen quality in an Italian cross sectional study. Basic and clinical andrology. 2017;27(1):1-6.

[24] Agarwal A DD. Are men talking their reproductive health away? . Asian J Androl. 2015;17:433-4.

[25] Adams JA GT, Mondal D, Esteves SC, Mathews F. Effect of mobile telephones on sperm quality: a systematic review and meta-analysis. Environ Int. 2014;70:106-12.

[26] Liu K LY, Zhang G, Liu J, Cao J, Ao L, et al. Association between mobile phone use and semen quality: a systemic review and meta-analysis. . Andrology 2014;2:491-501.

[27] Nateghian Z, Aliabadi E. Aspects of environmental pollutants on male fertility and sperm parameters. Journalof Environmental Treatment Techniques. 2020;8(1):299-309.

[28] ST. T. Preventable causes of male infertility. World journal of urology. 1993 May 1;11(2):111-9.

[29] Pizzorno J. Environmental toxins and infertility. Integrative Medicine: A Clinician's Journal. 2018;17(2):8.

[30] Choy CM LC, Cheung LT, et al. . Infertility, blood mercury concentrations and dietary seafood consumption: A case-control study. BJOG 2002;109(10):1121-1125.

[31] Buck Louis GM SR, Schisterman EF, et al. . Heavy metals and couple fecundity, the LIFE Study. Chemosphere. 2012;;87(11):1201-1207.

[32] Burridge E. Bisphenol A: product profile. Eur Chem News. 2003;17:14-20.

[33] www.bisphenol-a.org. 2007.

[34] Vandenberg LN, Hauser R, Marcus M, Olea N, Welshons WV. Human exposure to bisphenolA (BPA). Reproductive toxicology. 2007;24(2): 139-77.

[35] YOKOTA H, IWANO H, ENDO M, KOBAYASHI T, INOUE H, IKUSHIRO S-i, et al. Glucuronidation of the environmental oestrogen bisphenol A by an isoform of UDP-glucuronosyltransferase, UGT2B1, in the rat liver. Biochemical Journal. 1999;340(2):405-9.

[36] Ma R, Sassoon DA. PCBs exert an estrogenic effect through repression of the Wnt7a signaling pathway in the female reproductive tract. Environmental Health Perspectives. 2006;114(6):898-904.

[37] Diamanti-Kandarakis E, Bourguignon J-P, Giudice LC, Hauser R, Prins GS, Soto AM, et al. Endocrine-disrupting chemicals: an Endocrine Society scientific statement. Endocrine reviews. 2009;30(4):293-342.

[38] Li D-k, Zhou Z-j, Miao M-h, He Y-h, Wang J-t, Ferber J, et al. Urine Bisphenol-a (BPA) Level in Relation to Semen Quality and Sexual Dysfunction. Epidemiology. 2011;22(1):S79-S80.

[39] Castellini C, Totaro M, Parisi A, D'Andrea S, Lucente L, Cordeschi G, et al. Bisphenol A and male fertility: Myths and realities. Frontiers in Endocrinology. 2020;11:353.

[40] Al-Hiyasat AS, Darmani H, Elbetieha AM. Effects of bisphenol A on adult male mouse fertility. European Journal of Oral Sciences. 2002;110(2):163-7.

[41] Salian S, Doshi T, Vanage G. Neonatal exposure of male rats to Bisphenol A impairs fertility and expression of sertoli cell junctional proteins in the testis. Toxicology. 2009;265(1-2):56-67.

[42] Tainaka H, Takahashi H, Umezawa M, Tanaka H, Nishimune Y, Oshio S, et al. Evaluation of the testicular toxicity of prenatal exposure to bisphenol A based on microarray analysis combined with MeSH annotation. The Journal of Toxicological Sciences. 2012;37(3):539-48.

[43] Dobrzyńska MM, Radzikowska J. Genotoxicity and reproductive toxicity of bisphenol A and X-ray/bisphenol Acombination in male mice. Drug and Chemical Toxicology. 2013;36(1): 19-26.

[44] Tiwari D, Vanage G. Mutagenic effect of Bisphenol A on adult rat male germ cells and their fertility. Reproductive Toxicology. 2013;40:60-8.

[45] Grami D, Rtibi K, Hammami I, Selmi S, De Toni L, Foresta C, et al. Protective action of *eruca sativa* leaves aqueous extracts against bisphenol a-caused in vivo testicular damages. Journal of Medicinal Food. 2020;23(6):600-10.

[46] Kazemi S, Bahramifar N, Moghadamnia AA, Jorsarae SGA. Detection of bisphenol A and nonylphenol in rat's blood serum, tissue and impact on reproductive system. Electronic Physician. 2016;8(8):2772.

[47] Li D-K, Zhou Z, Miao M, He Y, Wang J, Ferber J, et al. Urine bisphenol-A (BPA) level in relation to semen quality. Fertility and Sterility. 2011;95(2):625-30. e4.

[48] Xiao G, Wang R, Cai Y, He G, Zhou Z. Effect of bisphenol A on semen quality of exposed workers: a pilot study. Zhonghua lao dong wei sheng zhi ye bing za zhi= Zhonghua laodong weisheng zhiyebing zazhi= Chinese journal of industrial hygiene and occupational diseases. 2009;27(12): 741-3.

[49] Pollard SH, Cox KJ, Blackburn BE, Wilkins DG, Carrell DT, Stanford JB, et al. Male exposure to bisphenol A (BPA) and semen quality in the Home Observation of Periconceptional Exposures (HOPE) cohort. Reproductive Toxicology. 2019;90:82-7.

[50] Omran GA, Gaber HD, Mostafa NAM, Abdel-Gaber RM, Salah EA. Potential hazards of bisphenol A exposure to semen quality and sperm DNA integrity among infertile men. ReproductiveToxicology. 2018;81: 188-95.

[51] Adoamnei E, Mendiola J, Vela-Soria F, Fernández MF, Olea N, Jørgensen N, et al. Urinary bisphenol A concentrations are associated with reproductive parameters in young men. Environmental Research. 2018;161: 122-8.

[52] Ji H, Miao M, Liang H, Shi H, Ruan D, Li Y, et al. Exposure of environmental Bisphenol A in relation to routine sperm parameters and sperm movement characteristics among fertile men. Scientific Reports. 2018;8(1):1-9.

[53] Li J, Mao R, Zhou Q, Ding L, Tao J, Ran M-M, et al. Exposure to bisphenol A (BPA) in Wistar rats reduces sperm quality with disruption of ERK signal pathway. Toxicology Mechanisms and Methods. 2016;26(3):180-8.

[54] Chigrinets SV, Brukhin GV. Environmental Exposure to Endocrine Disruptor of Bisphenol A and Semen Quality of Men. Annals of the Russian Academy of Medical Sciences. 2018;73(5):338-43.

[55] Knez J, Kranvogl R, Breznik BP, Vončina E, Vlaisavljević V. Are urinary bisphenol A levels in men related to semen quality and embryo developmentafter medically assisted reproduction? Fertility and Sterility. 2014;101(1):215-21. e5.

[56] Pan D, Feng D, Ding H, Zheng X, Ma Z, Yang B, et al. Effects of bisphenol A exposure on DNA integrity and protamination of mouse spermatozoa. Andrology. 2020;8(2):96-486.

[57] Abou Ghayda R, Williams PL, Chavarro JE, Ford JB, Souter I, Calafat AM, et al. Urinary bisphenol S concentrations: Potential predictors of and associations with semen quality parameters among men attending a fertility center. Environment international. 2019;131:105050.

[58] Goldstone AE, Chen Z, Perry MJ, Kannan K, Louis GMB. Urinary bisphenol A and semen quality, the LIFE Study. Reproductive Toxicology. 2015;51:7-13.

Chapter 4

Pathological Conditons Related to Bisphenols and It's Compounds

Geethamani Palanisamy and Divya Palanisamy

Abstract

Bisphenols (BP) is one of the most important and highest volumes of chemicals produced in the universe. Each year, around 100 tons of bisphenol compounds are released into the atmosphere. In general, bisphenol is most widely used for production of polycarbonate (making plastic bottles like baby bottles and nursing products, dental sealants, CDs, DVDs, eye glasses, medical equipment's, plasticizers etc.) and polymeric resins (epoxy resins, impact resistant safety materials like sports goods etc.). Due to these unavoidable chemicals, human beings are affected by human chronic diseases like obesity, toxicity, neuro disorder, reproductivity disorders, diabetes, cardio related issues, birth defects, metabolic syndrome, breathing issues, digestive related issues, cancer, genetic mutation etc., Children are easily affecting due to the multi dose consumption of packed food containing BP (canned foods) than adults. Women are affecting polycystic ovaries due to the high-level deposition of BP.

Keywords: metabolic syndrome, bisphenols, obesity, toxicity, disruption of endocrine, disorders

1. Introduction to bisphenol compounds

The commercial production of Bisphenol compounds (BP) initiated by late 1950's, after the first epoxy resin was developed. A synthetically man-made chemical which is a polymeric monomer named bisphenol (BP) is widely used for the manufacture of plastic things and goods for the usage of daily life need for the human beings (food packages, drink containers, body lotions, playing toys, house hold plastic things, nursing products, decorators and water pipe lines, etc.) and industrial usages. Also, Bisphenol compounds are used for the manufacture of unsaturated polyester, polysulphones and polyetherimide. BP compounds of non-polymer are also used as an additive in flame retardants, thermal papers and brake fluids. The usage of BP is increasing more in more from last few decades in the universe, resulting BP is finding throughout the environment and also in human body [1] through their diet. A huge number of journals published based on the studies of BP and its compounds.

Chemically, BPA has two large phenyl groups with two electron rich hydroxyl group (alcohol and two methyl group). It forms lipophilic (associates with lipids), through the conjugation process, it makes a substance more water soluble. BPA is slightly more hydrophilic (associate with water), found in Adipose tissues and in breast milk too. The hydrophilic form is seen in urine and excrement. From the obtained information [2], BPA has a moderate potential for bioaccumulation and not found that to readily biodegrade.

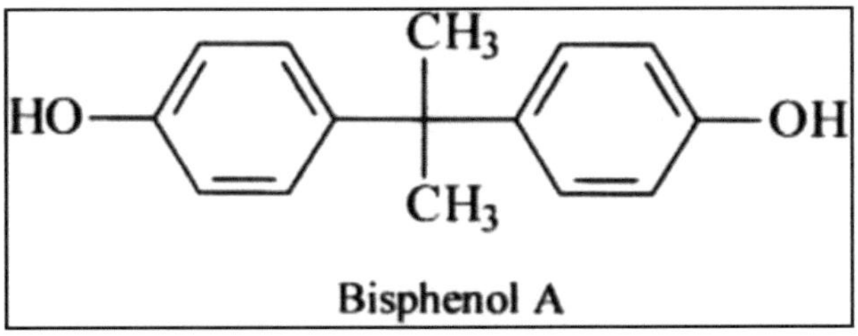

Figure 1.
Structure of BPA.

2. Bisphenol A

It was discovered by the Chemist A.P.Dianin in the year of 1891. These compounds are basically a carbon based synthesised compound belongs to the group of derivatives of diphenyl methane and bisphenols, which is colourless in nature called polycarbonate and are mostly stable and very strong in nature. The BPA components can withstand up to moderate to very high temperature even it is exposed to oven or furnace. Due to these properties, they can be used to manufacturing safety equipment's components, glassware, bullet proof windows, doors, etc. As one of the main component of epoxy resins in protective coatings or layers of those lining the inner surfaces of plastic tins or cans, BPA supposed to extend the shelf life of food and beverage products. **Figure 1** shows the structure of Bisphenol A. The toughness of BPA plastics has led to their use in medical equipment's like cardiopulmonary (heart-lung) machines, incubators, hemodialyzers (artificial kidneys) and dental sealants and dental fillers and their light weight and optical clarity glasses which has made for eyeglasses [3–5]. Also, the chemicals are found in a variety of other products, including compact discs (CD's) and other paper receipts.

3. Adverse health effects

In 1930s, the first studies indicated that, the BPA to be a weakly estrogenic molecule but later [6] confirmed that it has harmful effects through the animal research. The cancer like breast cancer, prostate cancer, Uro genital abnormalities (in Male babies), early onset of puberty in girls, metabolic disorders like Obesity and type-two diabetics, decreases in semen quality in men and neuro-behaviour problems including attention deficit hyperactivity disorder etc. are the possible diseases and disorder of BPA from the exposures during the critical periods.

4. Biological effects of bisphenol A

During 20th century, it was found it in only plastics even though scientists had developed BFA in 1930's as a man-made estrogens and its cancer causing (Carcinogenic) properties. The American endocrinologist led by his team in the early 1990's, unexpectedly found out, the BPA growth is medium in polycarbonate flask which is used to culture yeast cells. Further, they proceeded to isolate BP samples from the water in the flask and had been autoclaved, where they confirmed the chemical which was found same in the earlier detection (during 1930's). They also confirm that, BPA produced estrogenic effects in cells at the level of 5–10 times lower than who used for safety assessments companies where polycarbonate plastics are manufactured [7].

The leached plastics, resins in tin cans contains BPA products by various conditions including the photochemical break down, exposure of various temperature range (Low to high), maturity of plastics cans and/or resins and the presence of ethanol. In the middle of 1990's, number of studies confirms that, the main adverse effect due to BPA was reproductive system and development in animals by the interfering with their endocrine systems (energy balance and stress response) by the exposure level of BPA (both high and low level). The studies confirm that, due to the accumulation of BPA, it retards sexual behaviour in animals [8–10]. Also, it has been identified that the crossed placental barrier in animals (mammals) like mice and rats has been detected in human beings maternal and fetal serum which was also coincident with in human placental tissues. Thus, Bisphenol compounds found its way into tissues and fluids in the human womb. The chemical reaction attack and its effects in human fetal development is still not-clear. Similarly, the function of the human endocrine system is a matter to discuss. Much more speculation centres on whether BPA is a true endocrine disruptor chemical (EDC) in humans. The substituted Endocrine disruptor like DichloroDiphenylTrichloroEthane (DDT) & diethylstilbestrol, had been combined with birth defects, reduced fertility (infertility), and diseases such as obesity, diabetes, and carcinoma in humans. Derivatives of Bisphenol compounds (BPA, BPS and BPF) are used as alternatives to BPA, are associated with obesity, particularly in children [11, 12].

5. BPA with in the environment

From the industries like chemical, plastics coat and staining manufactures, paper mills or material recycling companies, foundries (casting sand) or any direct or indirect leaching from the above and landfills (waste metal dumping), BPA might enter in to the environment directly. The accumulation of BPA, totally affects the growth, reproduction and life time of aquatic organisms. The United States Environmental Protection Agency (EPA) reported in 2010 that more than 1,000,000 pounds (454,000 kilogrammes) of BPA were released into environmental reservoirs each year, including soil, rivers, lakes, and oceans. Leaching from landfills and release from municipal water supplies, such as those associated with wastewater-treatment plants and paper mills, are the primary sources of environmental contamination. Plastic pollution is a major source of BPA in the world's oceans. Despite the fact that seawater accelerates the breakdown of BPA plastics, the likelihood of leached BPA accumulating in the tissues of marine species is quite low. On the other hand, studies on terrestrial and freshwater species have shown that even low concentrations of the chemical can cause abnormalities when exposed for an extended period of time. BPA exposure, for example, causes an increase in micronuclei in root tip cells, indicating DNA damage in plants. BPA exposure causes sex ratios to become biased toward females in certain species of reptiles whose sex determination is normally influenced by temperature [13–16].

6. Effects of BP in human body

6.1 Neurotoxic, neuro behavioural and its effects

The developmental exposure of BP & BPA are does not appear to affects the sensory system, the spontaneous or Laboratory animals' self-activity or sexual behaviour. At dietary doses below 5 mg/kg bw per day, changes in brain biochemical signalling, morphometric and cellular end-points within sexually dimorphic anatomical structures, and neuro-endocrine end-points were described. The most significant restriction is that methodological flaws cause uncertainty in the interpretation of results. Changes in anxiety and convergence of structural brain sex differences were identified as end-points suggestive of effects with possible human relevance based on the available data, although more research is needed to clarify uncertainties [17].

6.2 Cardiovascular effects

The toxicological evidence suggests that BPA has no discernible effect on cardiovascular function. The expert meeting is aware of upcoming cardiovascular function research that will soon inform judgements about cardiac end-points [18].

6.3 Metabolic disorders

Metabolic diseases are a new field of study, and the evidence currently available is insufficient to draw any conclusions about the possible harm to humans. However, the present evidence suggests that more research into the effects of BPA on adiposity, glucose or insulin control, lipids, and other diabetes or metabolic syndrome end-points is needed [19].

6.4 Effects on child and infants

Generally, the conservative assumptions made by the estimated international exposures reported are higher than comparable national estimates. The average and main exposure of exclusively breastfed babies (infants 0–6 months) to BPA was 0.3 μg/kg/day and exposure at the 95% was 1.3 μg/kg/day. When solid foods are introduced, exposure to BPA reduces after 6 months (at 6–36 months). For formula-fed newborns, there is a wide range of exposure estimates. Infants (0–6 months) fed liquid formula have a higher exposure than infants fed powdered formula, and infants fed polycarbonate (PC) bottles have a higher exposure than infants fed non PC bottles [20–23].

Infants (0–6 months) who are fed liquid formula out of PC bottles have the highest estimated exposure are 2.4 μg/kg/day and 4.5 μg/kg /day at the 95th percentile. For children older than 3 years, highest exposure estimates did not exceed 0.7 μg/kg / day and 1.9 μg/kg /day at the optimum. For adults, highest exposure estimates did not exceed 1.4 μg/kg/day and 4.2 μg/kg bw/day at the maximum.

For most subgroups evaluated, exposure to BPA through non-food sources is at least one order of magnitude lower than that from food, based on the limited data available. Food, on the other hand, is by far the most significant source of overall BPA exposure in the majority of demographic groups. In addition, possible sources of exposure have been identified (unpackaged food and thermal paper). However, due to a lack of data, researchers were unable to produce exposure estimates. BPA concentrations in unpackaged foods and data on the consumer use patterns for materials and products containing BPA, including specific geographical differences; and the contribution of dermal exposure to overall exposure are furnished from the data over the exposure of BPAs [24–29].

6.5 Some studies on BPA and obesity

The studies of Serbian involve the 103 women aged, 19–50 years measured BPA in first morning urine and the number of anthropometric measures including height, weight, and waist and circumference (WC) were collected. Milosevic et al.,

S.No	Particulars	Report
1	less than 18.5 kg/m^2	underweight
2	between 18.5 and 24.9 kg/m^2	normal
3	between 25 and 29.9 kg/m^2	is overweight
4	between 30.00 and 34.99 kg/m^2	class 1 obese
5	35.00 and 39.9 kg/m^2	class 2 obese
6	above 40 kg/m^2	class 3 obese

Table 1.
The diagnosis of obesity (WHO., 2000).

described a positive suggestion between BPA and obesity [30]. However, limitations of this investigation were cross-sectional sample collection and the quantities of participants were very small. Also, there is no physical activity data were collected. The recent study in USA, involves 977 adult women were conducted; where BPA (urine) were monitored, anthropometric measures were collected (including weight and height). The recent study of BPA (urine) of children and pregnant women were also determined in USA [31]. Of these 408 children were 3 years, 518 children where 5 years were monitored until 7 years of age, along with 369 pregnant women who's between the ages 18 and 35. The anthropometric measures consists of Fat mass index (FMI), body fat (BF) and WC were collected.

The study was to monitor the mothers and their children at different stages of their development. In this investigation, BPA concentration of pregnant women had a positive suggestion with FMI, BF and WC of children at age of 7 but not associated with birth mass and childhood body mass index z-scores (BMIZ) at age of 5 and 7 and there are changes in BMIZ from ages of 5 to 7. The physical activity information of participants was not provided in the limitation of this study. A study in China involving 1326 students aged between 9 and 12 also measured (BPA) urine where anthropometric measures were collected with weight, height, WC, hip circumference and skinfold thickness [32]. From this study, it shows that the BPA had positive relationship with obesity in girls but not in boys.

6.6 Obesity diagnosis

Generally, obesity can be defined by using body mass index (BMI) by WHO to identify the obesity in people. The diagnosis of obesity is represented in the **Table 1.** The child obesity is studied by the nomogram technique. If, BMI equal to or greater than the age- and gender-specific, the 95th percentile is considered as obese (Centre for disease control) [33–35]. An obese person accumulates excess BF in his or her muscle, bone, fat and water. Obese people were facing many health problems at high risk including hypertension, mortality, low high-density lipoprotein cholesterol or high or low-density lipoprotein cholesterol and high levels of triglycerides (dyslipidaemia), coronary heart disease, diabetes (Type II), osteoarthritis, gallbladder disease, stroke and some cancers including endometrial, breast, colon, kidney, and liver cancer and gallbladder [36–40].

7. Effects of exposure to BPs

There is only inadequate information about the adverse effects of non-BPA. However, it is believed that they have similar effects to BPA [41]. In human fluids or tissues including placental tissue, serum, foetal plasma and breast milk, the concentration of BPA has been determined. Many studies have been focussed on children and pregnant women, where high BPA levels were linked with chromosomal abnormalities and miscarriages and infertility in women and abnormal karyotypes in foetuses [42]. The high BPA levels causes to more unilateral or bilateral blood-filled ovarian bursae in women.

7.1 Effect of BPA in biota

In comparison to non-biotic and biotic environmental compartments, biota contains a small amount of ambient BPA. BPA's published bio-concentration factor (BCF) values are much below 1000, which the US Environmental Protection Agency deems to be the threshold for concern. BCFs for fish exposed to BPA have been reported to be quite low [32].

7.2 Effect of BP on wild life

Numbers of challenges are facing due to the exposure of BPA (high concentration) on wildlife now days. The complexities in the natural system including chemical mixture, spatial varying exposure levels with tropic interactions and related few studies investigated results, the effect of chemical exposure on wildlife in-situ [43]. Many BPA toxicity studies have been used endocrine related measurement end-points which triggered by other toxicological modes of action that was identifying these mechanisms may/may not be necessary in order to characterise the response to the environmental toxicity [44].

8. Relevance of the study to BFA

BPA metabolism takes place by glucuronidation once in the body, under the catalytic action of the enzymes. While uridine 5-diphospho-glucuronosyltransferase (UGT) catalyses the conversion of BPA-to-BPA glucuronide, sulfotransferase catalyses the conversion of BPA- to the BPA- sulphate. Both metabolites are very soluble and removed from the human body in urine. The biotransformation of BPF and BPS is still unclear, but reactions carried out in vivo and in vitro organisms indicate that BPF metabolism is similar to BPA, while published studies on the biodegradation of BPS are extremely scarce [45].

In response to the same negative health effects of BPA, the US Food and Drug Administration (FDA) banned the use of BPA in baby bottles, sippy cups, and infant formular containers in 2012 [46]. Obesity increases the risk of a number of debilitating and fatal diseases, including diabetes, heart disease, and some cancers (US National Heart, Lung and Blood Institute, 1998). Obesity reduces a person's quality and length of life, raises an individual's healthcare costs, and raises the health costs of a country with a high prevalence of obesity (US National Heart, Lung and Blood Institute, 1998). Obesity is caused by a variety of factors, including lifestyle, genetics, and the consumption of processed foods high in fat, sugar, or carbohydrate; however, BPA and analogues when ingested have been linked to obesity [47–51]. The causes of obesity are plenty, such as lifestyle, genetics, the eating of processed food rich in fat and sugar or carbohydrate; however, BPA and analogues when absorb into the human body play a role in promoting adipogenesis and cause weight gain resulting in obesity especially in adolescent [52–57].

9. Prevention measures

For developing safer replacement for the use of plastics, the following move can takes place against the use of BPA contained products. These steps may reduce the exposures,

- Motivate the manufacturers are creating more and more BPA-free products. Look for products labelled as BPA-free products. If a product is not labelled, avoid to buy.

- Avoid heating the plastic containers in oven and in the direct sunlight. It may cause breakdown the BPA molecule and leach to the food products.

- Reduce the usage of canned foods.

- Cut down the used cans

- Instead of using these products, go with alternates such as glass, porcelain, stainless steel, copper containers and earthen pots for hot foods as well as cold foods.

10. Conclusions

Many research studies suffer from design and analysis flaws, limiting their utility for this purpose. The biological significance of many of the more sensitive end-points is still debated, as is whether studies that only examined conventional end-points are adequate for detecting all potentially relevant effects. Few clear trends have emerged from studies of BPA's effects on wildlife. Terrestrial wildlife is likely to be exposed to low levels of BPA, and few studies have looked at environmentally relevant doses. Although the majority of BPA regulation focuses on human exposure through food packaging, these applications account for only a small portion of BPA use. In the absence of new regulations, if current trends continue, BPA production and environmental release will increase. BPA would not necessarily result in a safer or more thoroughly researched chemical substitute. A more cautious approach to chemical regulation and use may reduce potential environmental impacts. Issues like these will continue to arise as humans become more reliant on chemical advances to meet global needs.

Author details

Geethamani Palanisamy* and Divya Palanisamy
Department of Chemistry, KGISL Institute of Technology,
Coimbatore, Tamilnadu, India

*Address all correspondence to: drpgeethamani@gmail.com

References

[1] Apau J, Acheampong A, Adua E. Exposure to bisphenol A, bisphenol F, and bisphenol S can result in obesity in human body. Medicinal Chemistry. 2018;**4**:1-8

[2] Available from: https://www.healthandenvironment.org/environmental-health/environmental-risks/chemical-environment-overview/bpa

[3] Baillie-Hamilton PF. Chemical toxins: A hypothesis to explain the global obesity epidemic. The Journal of Alternative & Complementary Medicine. 2002;**8**(2):185-192

[4] Bonefeld-Jorgensen EC, Long M, Hofmeister MV, Vinggaard AM. Endocrine-disrupting potential of bisphenol A, bisphenol A dimethacrylate, 4-nnonylphenol, and 4-n-octylphenol in vitro: New data and a brief review. Environmental Health Perspectives. 2007;**115**:69. DOI: 10.1289/ehp.9021

[5] Cabaton N, Zalko D, Rathahao E, Canlet C, Delous G, Chagnon MC, et al. Biotransformation of bisphenol F by human and rat liver subcellular fractions. Toxicology In Vitro. 2008;**22**(7):1697-1704. DOI: 10.1016/j.tiv.2008.07.004

[6] Casals-Casas C, Desvergne B. Endocrine disruptors: From endocrine to metabolic disruption. Annual Review of Physiology. 2011;**73**:135-162. DOI: 10.1146/annurev-physiol-012110-142200

[7] Clark E. Sulfolane and sulfones. Kirk-Othmer encyclopedia of chemical technology. Composition, H. B. (1987). In: Growth, Aging, Nutrition and Activity. New York: Springer-Verlag; 2012

[8] Danzl E, Sei K, Soda S, Ike M, Fujita M. Biodegradation of bisphenol A, bisphenol F and bisphenol S in seawater. International Journal of Environmental Research and Public Health. 2009;**6**(4):1472-1484. DOI: 10.3390/ijerph6041472

[9] Baillie-Hamilton PF. Chemical toxins: A hypothesis to explain the global obesity epidemic. The Journal of Alternative & Complementary Medicine. 2002;**8**(2):185-192

[10] Inadera H. Neurological Effects of Bisphenol A and its Analogues. International Journal of Medical Sciences. 2015;**12**(12):926-936. DOI: 10.7150/ijms.13267

[11] Bonefeld-Jorgensen EC, Long M, Hofmeister MV, Vinggaard AM. Endocrine-disrupting potential of bisphenol A, bisphenol A dimethacrylate, 4-nnonylphenol, and 4-n-octylphenol in vitro: New data and a brief review. Environmental Health Perspectives. 2007;**115**:69. DOI: 10.1289/ehp.9021

[12] Cabaton N, Zalko D, Rathahao E, Canlet C, Delous G, Chagnon MC, et al. Biotransformation of bisphenol F by human and rat liver subcellular fractions. Toxicology In Vitro. 2008;**22**(7):1697-1704. DOI: 10.1016/j.tiv.2008.07.004

[13] Casals-Casas C, Desvergne B. Endocrine disruptors: From endocrine to metabolic disruption. Annual Review of Physiology. 2011;**73**:135-162. DOI: 10.1146/annurev-physiol-012110-142200

[14] Clark E. Sulfolane and sulfones. Kirk-Othmer encyclopedia of chemical technology. Composition, H. B. (1987). In: Growth, Aging, Nutrition and Activity. New York: Springer-Verlag; 2012

[15] Danzl E, Sei K, Soda S, Ike M, Fujita M. Biodegradation of bisphenol A, bisphenol F and bisphenol S in

seawater. International Journal of Environmental Research and Public Health. 2009;**6**(4):1472-1484. DOI: 10.3390/ijerph6041472

[16] Williams EP, Mesidor M, Winters K, Dubbert PM, Wyatt SB. Overweight and obesity: Prevalence, consequences, and causes of a growing public health problem. Current Obesity Reports. 2015;**4**:363-370

[17] Yamada H, Furuta I, Kato EH, Kataoka S, Usuki Y, Kobashi G, et al. Maternal serum and amniotic fluid bisphenol A concentrations in the early second trimester. Reproductive Toxicology. 2002;**16**(6):735-739

[18] Yokota H, Iwano H, Mari E, Kobayashi T, Inoue H, Ikushiro S-I, et al. Glucuronidation of the environmental oestrogen bisphenol A by an isoform of UDP-glucuronosyltransferase, UGT2B1, in the rat liver. Biochemical Journal. 1999;**340**(2):405-409

[19] Milosevic M et al. Immunoglobulins G from sera of amyotrophic lateral sclerosis patients induce oxidative stress and upregulation of antioxidative system in BV-2 microglial cell line. Frontiers in Immunology, Multiple Sclerosis and Neuroimmunology. 2017;**2017**(8):1619. DOI: 10.3389/fimmu.2017.016191-15

[20] Song Y, Hauser R, Hu F, Franke A, Liu S, Sun Q. Urinary concentrations of bisphenol A and phthalate metabolites and weight change: A prospective investigation in US women. International Journal of Obesity. 2014;**38**(12):1532-1537. DOI: 10.1038/ ijo.2014.63

[21] Suiko M, Sakakibara Y, Liu M-C. Sulfation of environmental estrogen-like chemicals by human cytosolic sulfotransferases. Biochemical and Biophysical Research Communications. 2000;**267**(1):80-84

[22] US Food and Drug Administration (FDA). CFR part 177. Indirect Additives Polymers Final Rule Federal Register. 2012;**77**:41899-41902

[23] Food US, Administration D. Bisphenol A (BPA): Use in Food Contact Application. U.S. Department of Health and Human Services, Food and Drug Administration; 2012 Retrieved June 26, 2012 from http://www.fda.gov/NewsEvents/PublicHealthFocus/ucm064437.htm

[24] U.S. Food and Drug Administration. Summary of Bisphenol A Biomonitoring Studies. Washington, DC: U.S. Department of Health and Human Services, Food and Drug Administration; 2009. Memorandum from V. Komolprasert, dated November 16, 2009. http://www.regulations.gov/#!documentDetail;D=FDA-2010-N0100-0010

[25] US National Heart, Lung and Blood Institute. (1998). Clinical guidelines on the identification, evaluation and treatment of overweight and obesity in adults. The Evidence Report. United States. Retrieved May 13, 2010 from http://www. nhlbi. nih. gov/guidelines/obesity/prctgd_c. pdf

[26] National Toxicology Program. NTP-CERHR Monograph on the Potential Human Reproductive and Developmental Effects of Bisphenol A. Research Triangle Park, NC: National Institute of Environmental Health Sciences, National Toxicology Program; 2008 http://ntp.niehs.nih.gov/ntp/ohat/bisphenol/bisphenol.pdf

[27] Palanza PL, Howdeshell KL, Parmigiani S, vom Saal FS. Exposure to a low dose of bisphenol A during fetal life or in adulthood alters maternal behavior in mice. Environmental Health Perspectives. 2002;**110**(Suppl 3):415-422

[28] Rochester JR, Bolden AL. Bisphenol S and F: A systematic review and comparison of the hormonal activity of bisphenol A substitutes. Environmental

Health Perspectives (Online). 2015;**123**(7):643-650. DOI: 10.1289/ehp.1408989

[29] Rosenmai AK, Dybdahl M, Pedersen M, Alice van VugtLussenburg BM, Wedebye EB, Taxvig C, et al. Are structural analogues to bisphenol a safe alternatives? Toxicological Sciences. 2014;**139**(1):35-47

[30] Hoepner A et al. The Effects of Corporate and Country Sustainability Characteristics on The Cost of Debt: An International Investigation. Journal of Business Finance & Accounting. 2016;**43**(1):n/a-n/a. DOI: 10.1111/jbfa.12183

[31] Li J, Carlson BE, Lacis AA. A study on the temporal and spatial variability of absorbing aerosols using total ozone mapping spectrometer and ozone monitoring instrument aerosol index data. Journal of Geophysical Research. 2009;**114**:D09213. DOI: 10.1029/2008JD011278

[32] Flint S, Markle T, Thompson S, Wallace E. Bisphenol A exposure, effects, and policy: A wildlife perspective. Journal of Environmental Management. 2012;**104**(19):14

[33] Ying G-G, Kookana RS. Sorption and degradation of estrogen-like endocrine disrupting chemicals in soil. Environmental Toxicology and Chemistry. 2005;**24**:2640e2645

[34] Yoon Y, Westerhoff P, Snyder SA, Esparza M. HPLC-fluorescence detection and adsorption of bisphenol A, 17b-estradiol, and 17a-ethynyl estradiol on powdered activated carbon. Water Research. 2003;**37**: 3530e3537

[35] Yu C-P, Chu K-H. Occurrence of pharmaceuticals and personal care products along the West Prong Little Pigeon River in east Tennessee, USA. Chemosphere. 2009;**75**:1281e1286

[36] Zeng G, Zhang C, Huang G, Yu J, Wang Q, Li J, et al. Adsorption behavior of bisphenol-A on sediments in Xiangjiang River, Central-south China. Chemosphere. 2006;**65**:1490e1499

[37] Zhang S, Zhang Q, Darisaw S, Ehie O, Wang G. Simultaneous quantification of polycyclic aromatic hydrocarbons (PAHs), polychlorinated biphenyls (PCBs), and pharmaceuticals and personal care products (PPCPs) in Mississippi river water, in New Orleans, Louisiana, USA. Chemosphere. 2007;**66**:1057e1069

[38] Zoeller RT, Bansal R, Parris C. Bisphenol-A, an environmental contaminant that acts as a thyroid hormone receptor antagonist in vitro, increases serum thyroxine, and alters RC3/neurogranin expression in the developing rat brain. Endocrinology. 2005;**146**:607e612

[39] Flint S, Markle T, Thompson S, Wallace E. Bisphenol A exposure, effects, and policy: A wildlife perspective. Journal of Environmental Management. 2012;**104**:19-34

[40] Yamamoto TA, Yasuhara A, Shiraishi H, Nakasugi O. Bisphenol-A in hazardous landfill leachates. Chemosphere. 2001;**42**:415e418

[41] Yang FX, Xu Y, Wen S. Endocrine-disrupting effects of nonphenol, bisphenol A and p, p0-DDE on Rana nigromaculata tadpoles. Bulletin of Environmental Contamination and Toxicology. 2005;**75**:1168e1175

[42] Wilson MP, Schwarzman MR. Health policy: Toward a new US chemicals policy: Rebuilding the foundation to advance new science, green chemistry, and environmental health. Environmental Health Perspectives. 2009;**117**(8):1202e1209

[43] Crain et al. Chapel Hill bisphenol A expert panel consensus statement:

Integration of mechanisms, effects in animals and potential to impact human health at current levels of exposure. HHS Publications. 2007;**24**(2):131-138

[44] Wright-Walters M, Volz C, Talbott E, Davis D. An updated weight of evidence approach to the aquatic hazard assessment of Bisphenol A and the derivation a new predicted no effect concentration (Pnec) using a nonparametric methodology. Science of the Total Environment. 2011;**409**:676e685

[45] Witorsch RJ. Endocrine disruptors: Can biological effects and environmental risks be predicted? Regulatory Toxicology and Pharmacology. 2002;**36**:118e130

[46] Searcey D, Richtel M. Obesity was Rising as Ghana Embraced Fast Food. Then Came KFC. Manhattan, NY: The New York Times Company; 2017

[47] Nishikawa Y. Endocrine Disruptors Effects of Bisphenol A on Human Health. JMAJ. 2003;**46**(3):103-107

[48] Pellegrini M, Bulzomi P, Lecis M, Leone S, Campesi I, Franconi F, et al. Endocrine disruptors differently influence estrogen receptor beta and androgen receptor in male and female rat vsmc. Journal of Cellular Physiology. 2013;**229**(8):1061-1068. DOI: 10.1002/jcp.24530

[49] Ottawa, Canada. Toxicological and Health Aspects of Bisphenol A Report of Joint FAO/WHO Expert Meeting 2-5 November 2010 and Report of Stakeholder Meeting on Bisphenol. 2010

[50] Apau J, Acheampong A, Adua E. Exposure to bisphenol A, bisphenol F, and bisphenol S can result in obesity in human body Cogent. Chemistry. 2005;**4**(1):1506601. DOI: 10.1080/23312009.2018.1506601

[51] Hoepner LA, Whyatt RM, Widen EM, Hassoun A, Oberfield SE, Mueller NT, et al. Bisphenol A and adiposity in an inner-city birth cohort. Environmental Health Perspectives. 2016;**124**(10):1644. DOI: 10.1289/ehp.1409567

[52] Gerona RR, Woodruff TJ, Dickenson CA, et al. Bisphenol-A (BPA), BPA glucuronide, and BPA sulfate in midgestation umbilical cord serum in northern and central California population. Environmental Science & Technology. 2013;**47**: 12477-12485

[53] Mahalingaiah S, Meeker JD, Pearson KR, et al. Temporal variability and predictors of urinary bisphenol A concentrations in men and women. Environmental Health Perspectives. 2008;**116**:173-178

[54] Huang H, Leung LK. Bisphenol a downregulates CYP19 transcription in JEG-3 cells. Toxicology Letters. 2009;**189**(3):248-252

[55] Vandenberg LN, Hauser R, Marcus M, Olea N, Welshons WV. Human exposure to bisphenol A (BPA). Reproductive Toxicology. 2007;**24**(2):139-177. DOI: 10.1016/j.reprotox.2007.07.010

[56] Vinas, Watson. Bisphenol S disrupts extradiolinduced nongenomic signalling in a rat pituitary cell line: Effect on cell functions. Environmental Health Perspectives. 2013a;**121**:352-358. DOI: 10.1289/ehp.1205826

[57] WHO. Technical Report Series 894. In: 2000 World Health Organization (WHO) "Obesity Situation and Trends" "http://www.who.org" int. Geneva: World Health Organization; 2014

Chapter 5

Toxic Effects of Bisphenols: A Special Focus on Bisphenol A and Its Regulations

Pınar Erkekoğlu, Anil Yirün and Aylin Balci Özyurt

Abstract

Bisphenol A (BPA), which is an abundant chemical in the environment, is suggested to cause different toxic effects, including endocrine disruption, reprotoxicity, developmental toxicity, and neurotoxicity. Due to these effects, regulatory authorities have restricted the use of BPA in different consumer products, particularly in products used by children. These restrictions have led to researchers and plastic industry to find new and safer alternatives. Today, bisphenol F (BPF) and bisphenol S (BPS) are highly used although their toxic effects are less known. In the past years, several studies showed that these derivatives might also act as endocrine disruptors and cause toxic effects. BPA is a substance that is carefully monitored by regulatory agencies, and toxicological data are evaluated regularly. The alternatives, such as BPF and BPS, should also be monitored, and the regulations concerning their use in consumer products must be implemented soon. The increase in the number of studies on BPA and different bisphenols is very important in terms of obtaining new toxicological data and guiding regulatory institutions. This chapter will mainly focus on BPA, its toxicity, BPA alternatives, and regulations implemented by different American and European authorities.

Keywords: bisphenol derivatives, endocrine disruptor, bisphenol A, bisphenol F, bisphenol S, regulations

1. Introduction

Bisphenols are a large family of chemicals used to produce polycarbonate and epoxy resins. Bisphenols contain two phenolic rings linked by a bridge formed by carbon and other chemical structures. There are many different derivatives of bisphenols, and the capital letter after bisphenol is used to express the reactant atom/component within the molecule. For example, the reactant group is acetone in bisphenol A (BPA), formaldehyde in bisphenol F (BPF, 4,4′-dihydroxydiphenylmethane) and sulfur trioxide in bisphenol S (BPS, 4,4′-sulfonylbisphenol) [1, 2].

The most commonly used derivative of bisphenols is BPA. BPA is a compound that consists of two phenol rings linked by a methyl bridge containing two functional methyl groups. Bisphenol A (BPA) was first synthesized in 1905 by the condensation of phenol and acetone in the presence of acidic catalyst. BPA is generally used to harden plastics since the 1940s. In the early 1930s, the use of BPA as an artificial estrogen was considered. However, diethylstilbesterol (DES), a more potent estrogenic compound, was preferred to BPA in pharmaceutical use [3, 4].

BPA is being used in plastics for many years in combination with other chemicals. BPA-containing plastics are on the market since 1957. In 2003, 856,000 tons of BPA was produced. It was recorded that 72% was used in the production of polycarbonate plastics and 21% was used in the production of epoxy resin. In 2009, global production of BPA exceeded 2.2 million tons. In 2011, it was reported that ~5 million tons were produced [5]. It is estimated that its production will increase to 10.6 million tons by 2022 [6].

It is shown that BPA can leach from polycarbonate plastics, epoxy resins, and other products in contact with foods and beverages, resulting in continuous exposure of the general population. Especially food coating materials or food containers containing BPA lead to a high risk of human exposure. In addition, actions such as mechanical abrasion, rubbing, or exposure to high temperatures also cause an increased risk of BPA release from these materials [7].

2. Biotransformation of bisphenol A

After oral exposure to BPA, this compound is rapidly absorbed from the gastrointestinal tract and undergoes first-pass effect in liver and intestines [8]. On the other hand, it is reported that BPA does not undergo the first-pass effect and is excreted more slowly after inhalation or dermal exposure [9]. Following oral absorption, BPA is rapidly metabolized in the human liver mainly by cytochrome P450 enzymes (CYP2C18 and to a lesser extent by CYP2C19 and CYP2C9) [10]. BPA is converted to inactive glucuronide conjugates by phase II reactions in the liver and kidney. In the presence of high levels of BPA, the glucuronidation pathway becomes saturated and the sulfatation pathway becomes active. BPA glucuronide formation is mediated by uridine diphosphate glucuronosyltransferases (UGT). UGT enzyme activity is lower in newborns compared with adults. Therefore, since the main detoxification pathway for BPA in humans and many other species is mainly by glucuronidation, it can be suggested that early-life exposure to BPA may have more serious consequences than exposure in adulthood. BPA is mainly excreted by urine. The elimination half-life of BPA is approximately 2–6 h, and almost the entire compound is excreted in the urine in approximately 42 h. In a study conducted with a small number of volunteers, it was shown that 9.5% of BPA was excreted unchanged in the urine, 69.5% as BPA glucuronide conjugate, and 21% as BPA sulfate conjugate [11, 12].

3. Studies on the toxic effects of BPA

In vitro, *in vivo,* and human studies have shown that BPA can have a wide variety of adverse effects on human health. Among these effects, reproductive and development problems due to estrogenic and anti-androgenic effects of BPA (i.e., alterations in estrogen and/or testosterone levels, changes in semen quality, low birth weight), metabolic diseases (such as diabetes and obesity), thyroid hormone disorders, organ damage (possibly due to oxidative stress, epigenetic alterations, and direct toxic effect), cancer (breast, prostate, etc.), and neurotoxicity (behavioral disorders, changes in brain chemistry, neurological diseases/disorders) are highly studied, and BPA exposure is linked to different disorders by many scientists [13–15].

3.1 Reproductive toxicity

Bisphenols may affect both female and male reproductive health although their effects are suggested to be more pronounced in males. Recent human studies show that BPA exposure in adulthood is associated with decreased ovarian response, lower fertilization success and embryo quality, and polycystic ovary syndrome (PCOS). Moreover, BPA may cause male sexual dysfunction, decreased sperm quality, and changes in sex hormone concentrations. Both *in vitro* and *in vivo* studies indicate that environmental exposure to high doses of BPA may have adverse effects on reproductive health [13, 16, 17].

The harmful effect of BPA on male reproductive health can occur during embryonic and/or pubertal and/or adulthood. BPA may affect the hypothalamic-pituitary-testicular axis by modulating hormone synthesis, altering the expression and function of related receptors and disrupting testicular functions. Bisphenols, including BPA, are associated with reproductive disorders and infertility in males. In addition, BPA causes oxidative stress in testis and epididymis by inhibiting antioxidant enzymes and stimulating lipid peroxidation. BPA has been reported to have both estrogenic and anti-androgenic effects through interaction with estrogen (ER) and androgen receptors (AR) [18, 19].

3.2 Metabolic disorders

In the last 40 years, humans are abundantly exposed to wide variety of endocrine disrupting chemicals (EDCs) including bisphenols. Therefore, the first question that comes to mind is whether these diseases are associated with EDCs.

Many epidemiological studies associate EDCs, especially BPA, with obesity in humans. Most studies are cross-sectional analyses of the US National Health and Nutrition Examination Survey (NHANES) data in adults and children. The results of these research show that the higher the urinary BPA concentration, the higher the odds of obesity and larger waist circumference. Another study using a cohort in China reported an association between urinary BPA concentrations and overweight, obesity, insulin resistance, and diabetes mellitus. To our knowledge, only one prospective study has examined the association between prenatal and early-life exposure to BPA and children's body mass in 9-year-old girls. That work concluded that girls with the highest exposure to BPA *in utero* had lower weight for the same height than girls with the lowest exposure, a result that contradicts the previous studies. Due to such inconsistencies, further studies are required on larger sample sizes [20, 21].

Although pancreatic cells and adipocytes are not estrogen target tissues, they contain functional estrogen receptors (ERs). The insulin-increasing effect of BPA is similar to the effect of estrogen and occurs *via* ERα. Chronic hyperinsulinemia and subsequent insulin resistance have been observed in chronic administration of BPA [22].

3.3 Thyroid disruption

According to the results of the mechanistic studies, it has been stated that BPA can impair thyroid functions through many pathways. BPA has both agonistic and antagonistic effects on thyroid function as it can bind to thyroid receptors. It is suggested that BPA acts as a T_3 antagonist by binding to thyroid receptors with weak bonds and can inhibit transcriptional activity mediated by these receptors [23].

In a study conducted to examine the possible relationship between BPA exposure during pregnancy and thyroid hormone levels in the newborns and the mothers, urine samples were obtained from 476 women in the first and second trimesters of their pregnancies and their free and total T_4 and thyroid stimulating hormone (TSH) levels were measured. In addition, TSH levels were determined in newborns. Researchers stated that exposure to BPA during pregnancy might cause a decrease in total T_4 levels in pregnant women and significant decreases in TSH levels especially in male newborns [24].

3.4 Neurodevelopmental and neuroendocrine effects

In the recent years, studies showed that the exposure to EDCs was related to cognitive deficiencies, slow neurodevelopment, increases in the incidence of aggression and depression, hyperactivity, and attention deficit problems [25–27].

It is reported that EDCs can have a wide range of effects on brain development, and many different mechanisms are proposed. Some of these effects are suggested to be through the neuroendocrine system. The neuroendocrine system is a complex system consisting of neurons, glands, non-endocrine tissues, humoral signals, hormones, and neurochemicals that function to regulate physiological and behavioral processes. There is a growing evidence that antropogenic chemicals, such as EDCs, may act on the neuroendocrine system, and they may affect peripheral organ systems and physiological processes. Functions of neuroendocrine system are largely related to the functions of neurotransmitters. Evidence suggests that brain neurotransmitter systems (including dopaminergic, adrenergic, serotonergic, and cholinergic systems) play an important role in the activation and/or inhibition of neuroendocrine system. This relationship necessitates the examination of neurotransmitters for the evaluation of neuroendocrine system. The regulation of both dopamine and serotonin production by estrogen-dependent mechanisms makes these systems vulnerable to the adverse effects of EDCs. Previous studies have reported that BPA and phthalate exposure might lead to imbalance in the levels of these neurotransmitters in various regions of the brain [15, 28, 29].

3.5 Atopic diseases

Estrogen receptors are found in many immune regulatory cells. Not only endogenous estrogens, but also environmental estrogens (xenoestrogens) play a role in allergic reactions. Worsening of asthma symptoms is reported among women (30–40%) at certain times of the menstrual cycle. Estrogens can increase antigen-presenting cell function and immunoglobulin E (IgE) synthesis by B cells, both in turn can trigger allergic diseases. It also promotes degranulation of mast cells/basophils. Studies show that BPA exposure increases the risk and incidence of allergic diseases [30, 31].

4. Bisphenol derivatives as alternatives to bisphenol A

Due to its adverse effects on human health, regulations have limited the use of BPA in various products (bottle bottles, toys, food containers, thermal papers). This has led to the search for alternative substances to BPA. BPF and BPS are structurally similar to BPA and they are widely used in industrial products as alternatives [4, 6]. It is known that BPS has a very common use. According to the European Chemicals Agency (ECHA), 1000–10,000 million tons of BPS are produced or imported annually in Europe [32]. BPF is still a low-use chemical, at least in Europe when compared with BPA and BPS [4, 6].

The sources of exposure to BPA and its derivatives BPS and BPF are very similar worldwide. Humans are exposed to bisphenol derivatives orally through food, dermally with personal care products and thermal papers, and by inhalation of environmental dusts. BPA, BPF, and BPS have been detected in many environmental samples, including soil, sediments, water, and sewage sludge [4, 6]. In addition,

BPS and BPF have been detected in the content of many products, such as personal care products in daily use (e.g. body washes, hair care products, makeup, lotions, toothpaste) [33], paper products (e.g. currency, food cards, flyers, tickets, mailing envelopes, plane boarding), and foods (e.g. dairy products, meat and meat products, vegetables, canned foods, cereals) [4, 6]. BPS is also used in cleaning products, electrical product coatings, and various industrial applications as a component of phenolic resin, as well as in thermal papers, including products marketed as "BPA-free paper." BPF is present in systems requiring increased thickness and durability such as water pipes, dental sealants, tank and pipe coatings, industrial floors, road and bridge deck coatings, structural adhesives, and mortars (i.e., high solids/high build systems). Moreover, it is also used in food packaging. BPF is also a component of epoxy resins [4, 6].

Recently, BPS and BPF have attracted the attention of many researchers due to their increasing use. Numerous studies on BPF and BPS have contributed to the determination of their toxic effect profiles and have guided various regulations. Various *in vitro* and *in vivo* studies have shown that these substances may also show estrogenic activity similar to BPA and may have endocrine disrupting effects due to its effects on ERs, ARs, and thyroid hormone receptors. Studies have also shown that they might cause reproductive toxicity, cytotoxicity, genotoxicity, and mutagenicity [34–37].

5. Regulations on bisphenol A and its derivatives

5.1 Food and drug administration

Food and Drug Administration (FDA) banned the use of BPA in baby bottles and sippy cups in June 2012. Afterward, the FDA banned the use of BPA in food packages used in baby nutrition products in June 2013 [38]. FDA has set the oral "no observed adverse effect level (NOAEL)" value for BPA at 5 mg/kg bw/day [39].

5.2 European food safety authority

The European Food Safety Authority (EFSA) comprehensively reassessed BPA exposure and toxicity in January 2015 and reduced the tolerable daily intake (TDI) for BPA from 50 to 4 µg/kg body weight/day. EFSA stated that different evaluations will be made and that this is a temporary value. EFSA experts calculated the "benchmark dose" for BPA (in which BPA causes a small adverse effect in the kidneys of mice) as 8960 µg/kg bw/day. Considering the difference between species, this value has been calculated as 609 µg/kg bw/day for humans [40].

In 2020, two projects carried out by Belgium and ECHA on the toxic effects of BPS were completed. According to the results of these two studies, the oral NOAEL value was determined as 20 mg/kg/day in rats. It has been concluded that this value is not at a level to change the "specific migration level" (SML) (i.e., the amount of substance allowed to leak into the food), which is 0.05 mg/kg, and therefore, there is no risk of BPS in contact with food [41]. EFSA's scientists recommend that more toxicological data are needed for the safe use of BPS in food contact materials. They suggest that these data can clarify its possible use as an alternative to BPA [42].

The NOAEL value of BPS for developmental toxicity and developmental immunotoxicity was determined as 20 mg/kg bw/day [42]. While the NOAEL value for general systemic toxicity was 60 mg/kg body weight, a high value of 180 mg/kg bw/day was determined for developmental neurotoxicity, fertility, and reproductive disorders [42]. However, new data on the biotransformation of BPS support that

BPS is rapidly metabolized and eliminated from rats [42]. Therefore, EFSA recommends that more toxicological data should be collected in order to put new regulations on action for BPS [42].

5.3 European Commission

Bisphenol A is classified as a substance, which "may harm fertility (Repr. 1B)"; "cause respiratory tract irritation (STOT SE 3)"; lead to "to serious eye damage (eye damage 1)" and cause "skin allergies (skin sen. 1)" in the EU in 2008 [43]. On March 29, 2010, the Danish Government banned the use of BPA-containing food contact containers for children between 0 and 3 years of age. In July 2010, the Commission of the French Government and on July 9, 2010 all EU member States decided to implement the safeguards laid down in Article 18 of Regulation (EC) No 1935/2004 and to temporarily prohibit the importing, exporting, marketing, and manufacturing of baby bottles containing BPA. Therefore, it was stated that all BPA-containing baby bottles on the EU market should be replaced by mid-2011. With the Commission's updated opinion in 2011, the decision to ban the use of BPA in the production of polycarbonate baby bottles continues [44].

In EU, permissible migration limit values for chemicals used in chewable toys, which are used by children under the age of 3, are set within the scope of the "Toy Safety Directives." According to this directive, it states that the BPA content that can be found in toys should be lower than 0.04 mg/L [45].

By the regulations accepted in 2011, the specific migration limit (SML) was determined as 0.6 mg of BPA per kg of food. The opinion adopted in the EU on December 11, 2014 also defined sources of non-dietary exposure (airborne exposure, ingestion of dust, and ingestion through the skin because of contact with thermal paper and cosmetics). The panel concluded that exposure estimates to BPA through dietary and non-dietary sources were below the TDI and lower than levels that might lead to health effects for the highest-exposure groups, including infants, children, and adolescents [44].

In the EU, restrictions and regulations for food-contact plastics are also beginning to be applied to the use of BPA in the inner coatings and varnishes of non-plastic food containers. In particular, precautions should be taken for the coating materials used in baby and child products so that BPA does not migrate to this product. The SML level should not exceed 0.05 mg BPA per kg food. Therefore, producers should submit to the competent authorities appropriate supporting documents confirming the declaration of conformity. Varnished or coated materials and items that were legally released before September 6, 2018 are allowed to remain on the market until stocks last. The regulation is valid for productions after this date [46].

The classification of substances of very high concern (SHVC) by Registration, Evaluation, Authorization and Restriction of Chemicals (REACH) is based solely on the properties of the substance itself, without considering the potential risks associated with the use and exposure of the substance [47]. BPA is included in the REACH SVHC Candidate List. In April 2019, the German authorities presented the proposal to classify BPA as both acute and chronic hazard Category 1 for the aquatic environment [48]. At the initiative of the French authorities, the use of BPA in thermal paper has been evaluated. In their assessments, the ECHA Committees stated that the BPA used in thermal paper does not pose a risk to consumers, but has potential risks to the health of workers who process receipts [49]. As of January 2, 2020, a concentration limit of 0.02% (w/w) has been set for the use of BPA in thermal papers [49]. For BPS, in accordance with Regulation (EU) No. 10/2011, the SML value for use as a monomer in food contact plastic materials (FCM) is 0.05 mg per kg food currently [49].

5.4 BPA regulations predicted for the future

BPA is a substance that is carefully monitored by regulatory agencies, and toxicological data are evaluated regularly. In addition, alternatives to BPA, which are planned to be replaced in the industry due to its toxic effects, are also closely monitored regulatory authorities [50]. In this context, ECHA and EU Member States have started to evaluate data on a large group of bisphenols, such as BPA, BPS, BPF, and their derivatives, from the beginning of 2020. In addition, France and Sweden suggested that the use of these substances in the textile, leather, and fur industries should be restricted because they may cause dermal toxicity [49]. More than 1000 substances, including BPA and its derivatives, are covered by Skin Sens under Regulation 1272/2008 on Labeling and Packaging of Chemicals (CLP), and they were classified as Skin irrit 2 (causes skin irritation) and/or Skin corr. 1/1A/1B/1C (causes severe skin burns and eye damage) [51]. For this reason, it is suggested that the use of BPA and its derivatives will most likely face restrictions. The increase in the number of studies on BPA and different bisphenols is very important in terms of obtaining toxicological data and guiding regulatory institutions.

6. Conclusion

Although complete of ban of BPA in different consumer products seems to be impossible in the near future, new and safer alternatives of this substance should be synthesized. Although BPF and BPS were suggested to be safer, data from different *in vitro*, *in vivo,* and human studies show that they may also cause toxic effects. Therefore, regulations for the use of different bisphenol derivatives should be implemented, and new data on their different toxic effects should be evaluated. Although life is inevitable without plastics, their uses particularly in products used by susceptible populations, such as infants and children, should be restricted by regulatory authorities. In addition to the restrictions imposed by regulatory agencies, public awareness will make a great contribution to reducing the exposure of sensitive populations to common plasticizers such as bisphenols.

Conflict of interest

The authors declare no conflict of interest.

Author details

Pınar Erkekoğlu[1*], Anil Yirün[1,2] and Aylin Balci Özyurt[1]

1 Faculty of Pharmacy, Department of Toxicology, Hacettepe University, Ankara, Turkey

2 Faculty of Pharmacy, Department of Toxicology, Çukurova University, Adana, Turkey

*Address all correspondence to: erkekp@yahoo.com

References

[1] Vandenberg LN, Maffini MV, Sonnenschein C, Rubin BS, Soto AM. Bisphenol-A and the great divide: A review of controversies in the field of endocrine disruption. Endocrine Reviews. 2009;**30**(1):75-95. DOI: 10.1210/er.2008-0021

[2] Eladak S, Grisin T, Moison D, Guerquin MJ, N'Tumba-Byn T, Pozzi-Gaudin S, et al. A new chapter in the bisphenol A story: Bisphenol S and bisphenol F are not safe alternatives to this compound. Fertility and Sterility. 2015;**103**(1):11-21. DOI: 10.1016/j.fertnstert.2014.11.005

[3] Vandenberg LN, Hauser R, Marcus M, Olea N, Welshons WV. Human exposure to bisphenol A (BPA). Reproductive Toxicology. 2007;**24**(2):139-177. DOI: 10.1016/j.reprotox.2007.07.010

[4] Rochester JR. Bisphenol A and human health: A review of the literature. Reproductive Toxicology. 2013;**42**:132-155. DOI: 10.1016/j.reprotox.2013.08.008

[5] Kang JH, Kondo F, Katayama Y. Human exposure to bisphenol A. Toxicology. 2006;**226**(2-3):79-89. DOI: 10.1016/j.tox.2006.06.009

[6] Lehmler HJ, Liu B, Gadogbe M, Bao W. Exposure to bisphenol A, bisphenol F, and bisphenol S in U.S. adults and children: The National Health and nutrition examination survey 2013-2014. ACS Omega. 2018;**3**(6):6523-6532. DOI: 10.1021/acsomega.8b00824

[7] Rubin BS. Bisphenol A: An endocrine disruptor with widespread exposure and multiple effects. The Journal of Steroid Biochemistry and Molecular Biology. 2011;**127**(1-2):27-34. DOI: 10.1016/j.jsbmb.2011.05.002

[8] Ye X, Wong L-Y, Bishop AM, Calafat AM. Variability of urinary concentrations of bisphenol A in spot samples, first morning voids, and 24-hour collections. Environmental Health Perspectives. 2011;**119**(7):983. DOI: 10.1289/ehp.1002701

[9] Volkel W, Bittner N, Dekant W. Quantitation of bisphenol A and bisphenol A glucuronide in biological samples by high performance liquid chromatographytandem mass spectrometry. Drug Metabolism and Disposition. 2005;**33**(11):1748-1757. DOI: 10.1124/dmd.105.005454

[10] Nachman RM, Hartle JC, Lees PSJ, Grropman JD. Early life metabolism of bisphenol A: A systematic review of the literature. Current Environmental Health Reports. 2014;**1**(1):90-100. DOI: 10.1007/s40572-013-0003-7

[11] Völkel W, Colnot T, Csanády GA, Filser JG, Dekant W. Metabolism and kinetics of bisphenol A in humans at low doses following oral administration. Chemical Research in Toxicology. 2002;**15**(10):1281-1287. DOI: 10.1021/tx025548t

[12] Hanioka N, Naito T, Narimatsu S. Human UDP-glucuronosyltransferase isoforms involved in bisphenol A glucuronidation. Chemosphere. 2008;**74**(1):33-36. DOI: 10.1016/j.chemosphere.2008.09.053

[13] Tomza-Marciniak A, Stepkowska P, Kuba J, Pilarczyk B. Effect of bisphenol A on reproductive processes: A review of *in vitro*, *in vivo* and epidemiological studies. Journal of Applied Toxicology. 2017;**38**(1):51-80. DOI: 10.1002/jat.3480

[14] Benachour N, Aris A. Toxic effects of low doses of bisphenol-a on human placental cells. Toxicology and Applied Pharmacology. 2009;**241**(3):322-328. DOI: 10.1016/j.taap.2009.09.005

[15] Matsuda S, Matsuzawa D, Ishii D, Tomizawa H, Sutoh C, Nakazawa K.

Effects of perinatal exposure to low dose of Bisphenol A on anxiety like behavior and dopamine metabolites in brain. Progress in Neuro-Psychopharmacology and Biological Psychiatry. 2012; **39**(2):273-279

[16] Lassen TH, Frederiksen H, Jensen TK, Petersen JH, Joensen UN, Main KM, et al. Urinary bisphenol A levels in young men: Association with reproductive hormones and semen quality. Environmental Health Perspectives. 2014;**122**(5):478-484. DOI: 10.1289/ehp.1307309

[17] vom Saal FS, Cooke PS, Buchanan DL, Palanza P, Thayer KA, Nagel SC, et al. A physiologically based approach to the study of bisphenol A and other estrogenic chemicals on the size of reproductive organs, daily sperm production, and behavior. Toxicology and Industrial Health. 1998;**14**(1-2): 239-260. DOI: 10.1177/0748233798 01400115

[18] Takayanagi S, Tokunaga T, Liu X, Okada H, Matsushima A, Shimohigashi Y. Endocrine disruptor bisphenol A strongly binds to human estrogen-related receptor gamma (ERRgamma) with high constitutive activity. Toxicology Letters. 2006;**167**(2):95-105. DOI: 10.1016/j. toxlet.2006.08.012

[19] Acconcia F, Pallottini V, Marino M. Molecular mechanisms of action of BPA. Dose-Response. 2015;**13**(4):1-9. DOI: 10.1177/1559325815610582

[20] Carwile JL, Michels KB. Urinary bisphenol A and obesity: NHANES 2003-2006. Environmental Research. 2011;**111**:825-830. DOI: 10.1016/j. envres.2011.05.014

[21] Shankar A, Teppala S, Sabanayagam C. Urinary bisphenol A levels and measures of obesity: Results from the National Health and nutrition examination survey 2003-2008. ISRN Endocrinology. 2012;**2012**:965243. DOI: 10.5402/2012/965243

[22] Wang T, Li M, Chen B, et al. Urinary bisphenol A (BPA) concentration associates with obesity and insulin resistance. The Journal of Clinical Endocrinology and Metabolism. 2012;**97**(2):E223-E227. DOI: 10.1210/ jc.2011-1989

[23] Meeker JD, Calafat AM, Hauser R. Urinary Bisphenol A concentrations in relation to serum thyroid and reproductive hormone levels in men from an infertility clinic. Environmental Science & Technology. 2010;**44**(4):1458-1463. DOI: 10.1021/es9028292

[24] Chevrier J, Gunier RB, Bradman A, Holland NT, Calafat AM, Eskenazi B, et al. Maternal urinary bisphenol A during pregnancy and maternal and neonatal thyroid function in the chamacos study. Environmental Health Perspectives. 2013;**121**(1):138-144. DOI: 10.1289/ehp.1205092

[25] Honma T, Miyagawa M, Suda M, Wang RS, Kobayashi K, Sekiguchi S. Effects of perinatal exposure to bisphenol A on brain neurotransmitters in female rat offspring. Industrial Health. 2006;**44**(3):510-524. DOI: 10.2486/indhealth.44.510

[26] Inadera H. Neurological effects of bisphenol A and its analogues. International Journal of Medical Sciences. 2015;**12**(12):926-939. DOI: 10.7150/ijms.13267

[27] Landolfi A, Troisi J, Savanelli MC, Vitale C, Barone P, Amboni M. Bisphenol A glucuronidation in patients with Parkinson's disease. Neurotoxicology. 2017;**63**:90-96. DOI: 10.1016/j.neuro.2017.09.008

[28] Nakamura K, Itoh K, Yoshimoto K, Sugimoto T, Fushiki S. Prenatal and

Lactational exposure to low-doses of Bisphenol A alters brain monoamine concentration in adult mice. Neuroscience Letters. 2010;**484**(1):66-70. DOI: 10.1016/j.neulet.2010.08.021

[29] Yirun A, Ozkemahli G, Balci A, Erkekoglu P, Zeybek ND, Yersal N, et al. Neuroendocrine disruption by bisphenol A and/or di(2-ethylhexyl) phthalate after prenatal, early postnatal and lactational exposure. Environmental Science and Pollution Research International. 2021;**28**(21): 26961-26974. DOI: 10.1007/s11356-021-12408-9

[30] Whyatt RM, Rundle AG, Perzanowski MS, Just AC, Donohue KM, Calafat AM, et al. Prenatal phthalate and early childhood bisphenol A exposures increase asthma risk in inner-city children. The Journal of Allergy and Clinical Immunology. 2014;**134**(5):1195-1197. DOI: 10.1016/j.jaci.2014.07.027

[31] Zhou A, Chang H, Huo W, Zhang B, Hu J, Xia W, et al. Prenatal exposure to bisphenol A and risk of allergic diseases in early life. Pediatric Research. 2017;**81**(6):851-856. DOI: 10.1038/pr.2017.20

[32] EFSA. Assessment of new information on Bisphenol S (BPS) submitted in response to the Decision 1 under REACH Regulation (EC) No 1907/2006 [Internet]. 2019. Available from: https://www.efsa.europa.eu/en/supporting/pub/en-1844 [Accessed: 2021-11-12]

[33] Liao C, Kannan K. A survey of bisphenol A and other bisphenol analogues in foodstuffs from nine cities in China. Food Additives & Contaminants. Part A, Chemistry, Analysis, Control, Exposure & Risk Assessment. 2014;**31**(2):319-329. DOI: 10.1080/19440049.2013.868611

[34] Kose O, Rachidi W, Beal D, Erkekoglu P, Fayyad-Kazan H, Kocer Gumusel B. The effects of different bisphenol derivatives on oxidative stress, DNA damage and DNA repair in RWPE-1 cells: A comparative study. Journal of Applied Toxicology. 2020;**40**(5):643-654. DOI: 10.1002/jat.3934

[35] Yamasaki K, Noda S, Imatanaka N, Yakabe Y. Comparative study of the uterotrophic potency of 14 chemicals in a uterotrophic assay and their receptor-binding affinity. Toxicology Letters. 2004;**146**(2):111-120. DOI: 10.1016/j.toxlet.2003.07.003

[36] Lee S, Kim C, Shin H, Kho Y, Choi K. Comparison of thyroid hormone disruption potentials by bisphenols a, S, F, and Z in embryo-larval zebrafish. Chemosphere. 2019;**221**:115-123. DOI: 10.1016/j.chemosphere.2019.01.019

[37] Park C, Song H, Choi J, Sim S, Kojima H, Park J, et al. The mixture effects of bisphenol derivatives on estrogen receptor and androgen receptor. Environmental Pollution. 2020;**260**:114036. DOI: 10.1016/j.envpol.2020.114036

[38] US Food and Drug Administration (US FDA). 2018. Bisphenol A (BPA): Use in food contact application. [Internet]. Available from: https://www.fda.gov/food/food-additives-petitions/bisphenol-bpa-use-food-contact-application [Accessed: 2021-11-12]

[39] US Food and Drug Administration (US FDA). The FDA Bisphenol A Joint Emerging Science Working Group submits the following three memoranda with attachments as completion of the Working Group charge issued January 2011 and in response to FDA Science Board subcommittee recommendations of September 6, 2008. [Internet]. 2014. Available from: https://www.fda.gov/media/90546/download [Accessed: 2021-11-12]

[40] EFSA. Bisphenol A. [Internet]. 2017. Available from: https://www.efsa.europa.eu/en/topics/topic/bisphenol [Accessed: 2021-11-12]

[41] EFSA. Scientific Panel on Food Contact Materials, Enzymes and Processing Aids (CEP). [Internet]. 2019. Available from: https://www.efsa.europa.eu/sites/default/files/event/190522-m_1.pdf [Accessed: 2021-11-12]

[42] EFSA. Assessment of new information on Bisphenol S (BPS) submitted in response to the Decision under REACH Regulation (EC) No 1907/2006. [Internet]. 2020. Available from: https://efsa.onlinelibrary.wiley.com/doi/pdf/10.2903/sp.efsa.2020.EN-1844 [Accessed: 2021-11-12]

[43] Official Journal of the European Union. Regulation (Ec) No 1272/2008 Of The European Parliament And of The Council of 16 December 2008 on classification, labelling and packaging of substances and mixtures, amending and repealing Directives 67/548/EEC and 1999/45/EC, and amending Regulation (EC) No 1907/2006. [Internet]. 2008. Available from: https://eur-lex.europa.eu/legal-content/EN/TXT/?uri=celex%3A32008R1272 [Accessed: 2021-11-12]

[44] Official Journal of the European Union. Commission Directive 2011/8/EU of 28 January 2011 amending Directive 2002/72/EC as regards the restriction of use of Bisphenol A in plastic infant feeding bottles. [Internet]. 2011. Available from: https://eur-lex.europa.eu/legal-content/EN/TXT/?uri=CELEX%3A32011L0008 [Accessed: 2021-11-12]

[45] Official Journal of the European Union. Commission Directive (EU) 2017/898 of 24 May 2017 amending, for the purpose of adopting specific limit values for chemicals used in toys, Appendix C to Annex II to Directive 2009/48/EC of the European Parliament and of the Council on the safety of toys, as regards bisphenol A. [Internet]. 2017. Available from: https://eur-lex.europa.eu/legal-content/EN/TXT/PDF/?uri=CELEX:32017L0898&from=ES [Accessed: 2021-11-12]

[46] Official Journal of the European Union. Commission Regulation (EU) 2018/213 of 12 February 2018 on the use of bisphenol A in varnishes and coatings intended to come into contact with food and amending Regulation (EU) No 10/2011 as regards the use of that substance in plastic food contact materials. [Internet]. 2018. Available from: https://eur-lex.europa.eu/eli/reg/2018/213/oj [Accessed: 2021-11-12]

[47] European Chemicals Agency (ECHA). Proposals to identify substances of very high concern previous consultations. [Internet]. 2021. Available from: https://echa.europa.eu/proposals-to-identify-substances-of-very-high-concern-previous-consultations?diss=true&search_criteria_ecnumber=201-025-1&search_criteria_casnumber=77-40-7&search_criteria_name=4%2C4%27-%281-methylpropylidene%29bisphenol%3B+bisphenol+B [Accessed: 2021-11-12]

[48] The European Union. Bisphenol A. 2021. Available from: https://bisphenol-a-europe.org/regulatory-framework/european-legislation-on-chemicals/ [Accessed: 2021-11-12]

[49] European Chemicals Agency (ECHA). Bisphenol S has replaced bisphenol A in thermal paper. 2020. Available from: https://echa.europa.eu/fr/-/bisphenol-s-has-replaced-bisphenol-a-in-thermal-paper [Accessed: 2021-11-12]

[50] European Chemicals Agency (ECHA). Safer alternatives for

bisphenol A. 2021. Available from: https://echa.europa.eu/safer-alternatives-for-bisphenol-a [Accessed: 2021-11-12]

[51] European Chemicals Agency (ECHA). Guidance to Regulation (EC) No 1272/2008 on Classification, Labelling and Packaging of substances and mixtures. 2008. Available from: https://www.echa.europa.eu/documents/10162/23047722/draft_guidance_clp_hh_rac_forum_clean_en.pdf/85da9149-73e3-468b-b7bb-c2af5e5573e4 [Accessed: 2021-11-12]

Section 3

Detection Methods for Bisphenols

Chapter 6

Novel Sensor Based on Nanocarbon Transducer Functionalized by Iron (III) Porphyrin for the Impedimetric Detection of Bisphenol A

Zouhour Hsine and Rym Mlika

Abstract

In this chapter, an impedimetric response of iron (III) porphyrin ($Fe^{(III)}$TMPP) functionalized on gold transducer towards the detection of three phenolic compounds entitled bisphenol A (BPA), 2,2′-biphenol and catechol has been studied. The bisphenol A that has revealed the best affinity with $Fe^{(III)}$TMPP membrane has been chosen as the target analyte. For improved sensitivity of Au/$Fe^{(III)}$TMPP sensor towards BPA, a facile and efficient Au/RGO nanocarbon transducer based on reduced graphene oxide (RGO) has been prepared and used to support $Fe^{(III)}$TMPP membrane. The obtained Au/RGO/$Fe^{(III)}$TMPP structure was characterized by UV–visible (UV–vis) and electrochemical impedance spectroscopy (EIS) measurements, then applied as electrochemical platform for BPA detection. It has been discovered that the Au/RGO nanocarbon transducer has an amplified electron transfer kinetic compared to unmodified Au transducer. The Au/RGO/$Fe^{(III)}$TMPP structure has showed a better affinity towards BPA with a doubled sensitivity compared to that obtained with Au/$Fe^{(III)}$TMPP electrode. We demonstrated that the Au/RGO nanocarbon transducer not only enhances the electron transfer ability but also serves as a good template for the attachment of $Fe^{(III)}$TMPP through π- π interaction. This study reveals new high-potential of nanocarbon transducer based on RGO for the conception of electrochemical sensors with high sensitivity and short response time.

Keywords: iron (III) porphyrin, reduced graphene oxide, impedimetric sensor, nanocarbon transducer, bisphenol A

1. Introduction

Bisphenol A (BPA, 2, 2-bis (4-hydroxy phenyl) propane), is one of the most extensively used industrial compounds in the production of plastics due to its transparent, strong and light characteristics [1]. Till now, BPA has been widely employed as a monomer to synthesize polycarbonate, expoxy resin, polysulfone resin and other various polymer materials [2]. These polymer materials are mostly used to produce storage containers, nursing bottles, thermal papers, medical apparatus, food can linings and supply pipes [3]. However, toxicology studies have shown that BPA is a typical endocrine-disrupting compound (EDC) in which even a low level can mimic and interfere with hormonal activity by interfering with growth and reproductive development [4, 5]. Consequently, the popular use of BPA has raised serious concerns regarding its implications for food safety and environmental health. In fact, BPA can be released from waste plastics, thermal printing papers, compact disks, powder paints, and adhesives into food and water samples at low concentration (ppb level) and will eventually find its way into the human body [6]. Unsurprisingly, BPA was found to be present in many biological fluids such as human blood, serum, and urine [1]. Although many countries have begun to phase out the use of BPA [7], several of the BPA-containing products that often occupy landfills are still around. This means that BPA will continue to migrate into the environment through runoff and wastewater discharges, eventually contaminating our water resources and food supplies. Therefore, it is still needed to develop a sensitive and simple method for the determination of trace amounts of BPA in the environment. Notably, multiple procedures have been utilized for determining the contents of BPA in diverse matrices, including liquid chromatography-mass spectrometry [8], electrochemiluminescence, colorimetry, liquid chromatography coupled to UV/vis, fluorescence spectrometry, enzyme-linked immunosorbent assay (ELISA) [9], surface-enhanced Raman scattering (SERS) [10] and so forth. These methods can offer good accuracy and sensitivity, however they have some drawbacks, such as high-cost equipment, time consuming operation and unsuitability for onsite analysis [11, 12], thus restricting their application. On contrary, electrochemical sensors have been extensively used as an alternative solution for detecting trace levels of BPA due to their inherent advantages such as low cost, short analysis time, portability and excellent sensitivity [13]. Direct monitor BPA using an electrochemical sensor with a bare electrode has a poor response due to fouling and sluggish electron transfer kinetics [14]. In order to avoid and reduce this problem, several kinds of nanomaterials or their composites with excellent catalytic properties have been employed to modify the electrode. Amongst such materials, porphyrins and their derivatives have been long employed in electrochemical sensors applications [15] thanks to their special electrochemical properties [16]. These latter originated from the highly π-conjugated system of porphyrin which is an efficient platform for electron transfer [17]. Indeed, porphyrins are naturally occurring macrocyclic species that bind metals *via* nitrogen donor atoms on four pyrrole subunits, resulting in versatile chelating systems [18]. The coordination sites of porphyrin molecule can easily connected with metal ions such as Fe, Zn, Mg and so on to form stable metallo-porphyrins. This coordination increases the movement capacity of electrons [19], thus the electrocatalytic activity of the porphyrin. Among the metalloporphyrins, iron porphyrins have demonstrated excellent electrocatalysis for many biologically important target molecules [20] thanks to their electronic media role based on their reversible Fe(III)/Fe(II) redox states [21, 22]. Various carbon nanomaterials such as graphene and its derivates have been proven to be excellent carriers to enhance the sensitivity of sensors [23]. Graphene (or reduced graphene oxide, RGO), a 2D material with a single layer of an sp^2 carbon atom network densely packed in a honeycomb structure, has unique properties, such as large surface-to-volume ratio, high adsorption capacity, excellent conductivity and easiness of modifications [24]. This innovative nanocarbon material has been inserted into the sensitive membrane to form a nanocomposite as well as into the transducer to form a nanocarbon transducer. Recently, Nanocarbon Transducers based on RGO have enhanced the target analyte current response which makes them attractive for preparing highly sensitive sensors [25]. The aim of this chapter is to study the effect of nanocarbon transducer on the sensitivity of BPA sensor based on iron (III) porphyrin as a sensitive membrane.

2. Experimental procedure

2.1 Reagents

The triflato iron porphyrin ($Fe^{(III)}$TMPP) has been synthesized and characterized by proton NMR and FTIR according to the previously reported procedure [26]. The reduced graphene oxide (RGO) has been synthesized and characterized by FTIR and XPS as described previously [27]. Carbon nanotubes (MWCNTs) used in this study, have been obtained commercially from Baytubes, and produced in a high-yield catalytic process based on chemical vapor deposition (CVD). The diameter of these MWCNTs varies between 5 and 20 nm with a length of over 1 mm. Gold transducer (bare Au), indium tin oxide (ITO), phosphate-buffered saline tablets (PBS, pH = 7.4), acetone (≥99.5%), dimethylformamide (DMF, 99.8%), ethanol (≥99.9%), bisphenol A (BPA, ≥99%), catechol (≥99%) and 2,2′-biphenol (99%) were purchased from Sigma Aldrich (France).

2.2 Instruments and characterization methods

Electrochemical measurements were performed using an AUTOLAB PGSTAT 100 (supported by "FRA 4.9" software (Methrom)) coupled to a computer and an electrochemical cell (**Figure 1**). The electrochemical measurements were carried out in an electrochemical cell involving a three electrodes system purchased from BASi: bare Au (surface 2.01×10^{-2} cm^2) or modified Au with $Fe^{(III)}$TMPP or RGO/$Fe^{(III)}$TMPP membranes as the working electrode, Ag/AgCl (3 M KCl) as the reference electrode and platinum wire as the counter electrode. The analyses were performed by electrochemical impedance spectroscopy (EIS). The modified Au transducer is normally placed in a 0.1 M phosphate buffer solution (PBS (0.1 M), pH = 7) containing target species such as bisphenol A, 2,2′-biphenol and catechol

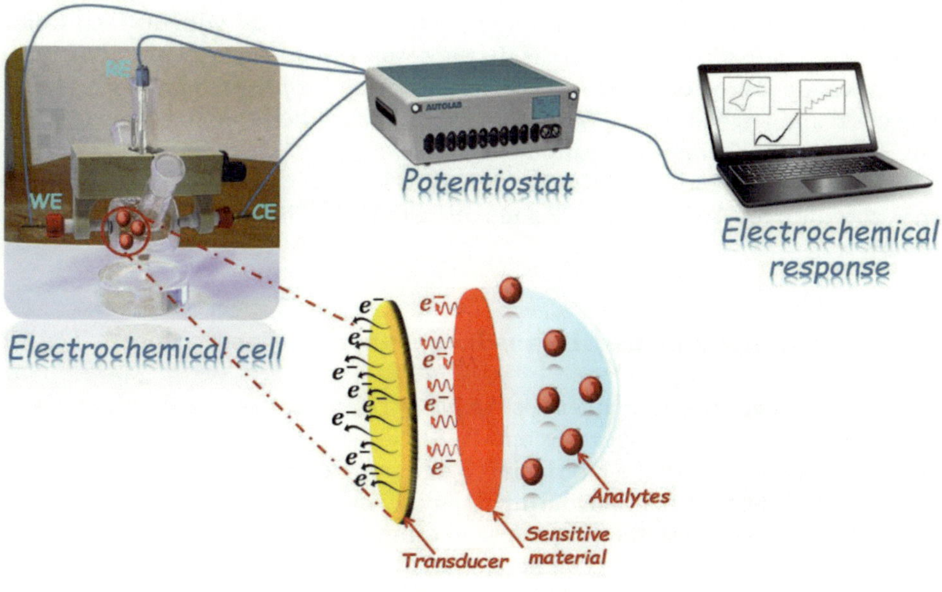

Figure 1.
Experimental electrochemical measurement device composed by electrochemical cell (place of electrochemical reactions between analytes and the sensitive membrane), potentiostat (electrochemical analysis system) and computer (electrochemical response display).

and then simply followed by fixing the potential. All experiments were conducted at ambient temperature (25°C).

EIS was measured at −0.9 V using an alternating potential of 10 mV amplitude in the frequency range from 100 kHz to 30 mHz.

The UV–vis spectra have been recorded with a Win ASPECT PLUS (validation for SPECORD PLUS version 4.2) spectrometer using a 100 μl quartz cell.

2.3 Preparation and measurement of electrochemical sensor

The used gold electrodes in this work have a dimension of 1 cm × 1 cm, where the thickness of the gold deposited by evaporation on Si/SiO_2 substrates is of the order of 50 nm [28]. Before the analysis, in order to improve the adhesion of the sensitive membrane on the electrode surface, the gold substrates were cleaned with acetone in an ultrasonic bath for 10 min and dried under nitrogen flow. Then, the gold substrate has been cleaned in piranha solution (1/3 H_2O_2 + 2/3 H_2SO_4) for about 2 min to activate the surface [29], after this treatment, the gold substrates were rinsed with ultra-pure water and dried under nitrogen flow.

For the preparation of Au/$Fe^{(III)}$TMPP sensor, the pretreated gold was drop-casted by 20 μL of $Fe^{(III)}$TMPP solution (4.7 mg in 500 μl DMF) and dried at 80°C in an oven for 1 h to evaporate residual solvent. The obtained modified electrode was then rinsed with distilled water to remove the non- attached $Fe^{(III)}$TMPP and dried under nitrogen flow.

The nanocomposites 2%CNTs/$Fe^{(III)}$TMPP and 4%CNTs/$Fe^{(III)}$TMPP were prepared by mixing 4.7 mg of $Fe^{(III)}$TMPP and different weight proportions of CNTs (2% and 4%) in 500 μl of DMF followed by sonication in an ultrasonic bath for 2 hours. Then, 20 μl of each nanocomposite solution was dropped onto the Au electrode, dried at 80°C in an oven for 1 h and rinsed with distilled water prior to electrochemical measurements.

For the construction of Au/RGO/$Fe^{(III)}$TMPP sensor, the preparation was divided into two steps. In the first step, the pretreated gold was drop-casted by 20 μL of RGO solution (1 mg in 1 ml DMF) and dried at 80°C in an oven for 1 h. The obtained Au/RGO nanocarbon transducer electrode was rinsed with distilled water to remove the non-adsorbed materials. In the second step, 20 μl of $Fe^{(III)}$TMPP solution was deposited onto the Au/RGO electrode by drop-casted method. After being dried and washed, the Au/RGO/$Fe^{(III)}$TMPP modified electrode was ready to be used for electrochemical measurements.

ITO/$Fe^{(III)}$TMPP and ITO/RGO/$Fe^{(III)}$TMPP electrodes were prepared using the same procedure for Au/$Fe^{(III)}$TMPP and Au/RGO/$Fe^{(III)}$TMPP sensors preparations respectively.

3. BPA sensor based on usual transducer functionalized by $Fe^{(III)}$TMPP

In order to check the attachment of the $Fe^{(III)}$TMPP on the bare Au electrode, electrochemical impedance spectroscopy (EIS) has been selected as a method of characterization thanks to the interfacial charge transfer properties that it can provide for the electrode surface during the modification process [30, 31].

Usually for EIS studies, the first step is to optimize the polarization potential by reducing the warburg diffusion component at low frequencies, which facilitates the interpretation of physico-chemical phenomena [32]. For our study, different negative potentials (E = −0.6 V, −0.7 V, −0.8 V and − 0.9 V) have been applied in a large frequency range (100 kHz to 30 mHz). We observe in **Figure 2** an obvious decrease of the half circle diameter correlated with the decrease of the applied

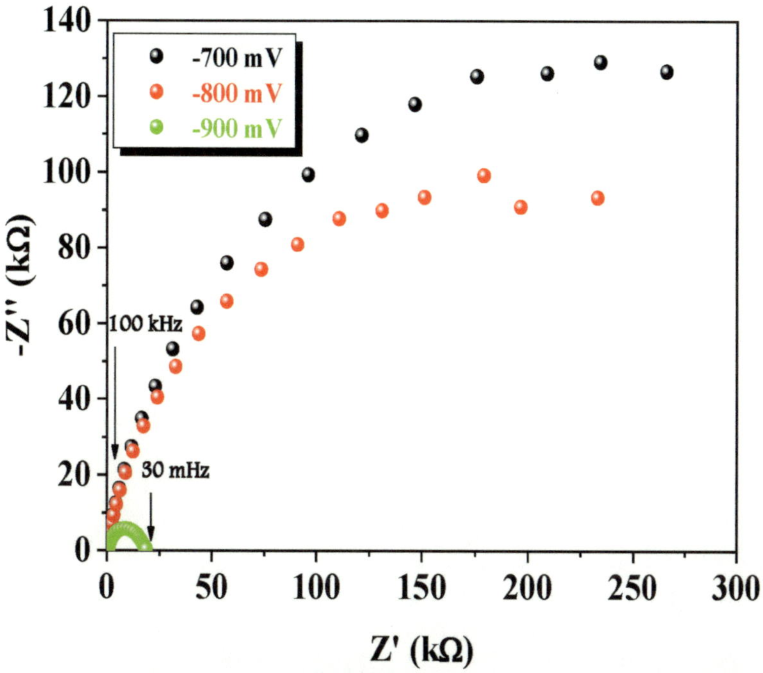

Figure 2.
Optimization of the polarization potential of Au/Fe$^{(III)}$TMPP electrode within a frequency range from 100 kHz to 30 mHz and an amplitude of 10 mV sinusoidal modulation in 0.1 M PBS (pH = 7).

potential. This decrease can be explained by the reduction of the charge transfer resistance as a function of the *dc* potential [33], which makes possible the observation of the kinetics of cations at the membrane/solution interface. As a result, we have chosen a continuous polarization of −900 mV throughout our next measurements.

Figure 3 shows the recorded Nyquist plots for bare Au before and after its modification by Fe$^{(III)}$TMPP membrane in a PBS solution without any additional external redox probe. The semicircle diameter is related to the charge transfer resistance (R_{ct}) of the electronic transfer from the porphyrin to the electrode [34]. Upon the modification of the Au transducer using Fe$^{(III)}$TMPP membrane, the semicircle diameter increased, which means the increase of R_{ct}. This is indicative of a better Au electrode surface coverage with Fe$^{(III)}$TMPP accompanied by the decrease in the electronic charge transfer.

The Nyquist diagram of Au/Fe$^{(III)}$TMPP electrode can be modeled by an equivalent electrical circuit formed by electrical components. This modeling is done thanks to a software "FRA2" which makes it possible to draw the proposed equivalent electrical circuit optimized by iteration. The choice of the latter is made according to the best fit which corresponds to the lowest value of the total error χ^2 as well as the error on each parameter. The values of the electrical components given for each Nyquist plot illustrate the electronic properties between the transducer/membrane/electrolyte interfaces which facilitate the interpretation of the electronic phenomena during the modification process.

In this study, the choice of the equivalent electric circuit was chosen based on the shape of the Nyquist diagram of the Au/Fe$^{(III)}$TMPP electrode as well as on its corresponding bode diagram (**Figure 4**). As can be seen in **Figure 4A**, the total impedance plot of the Au/Fe$^{(III)}$TMPP electrode has an enlarged shape. Consequently the Nyquist diagram of the modified electrode can be considered as an

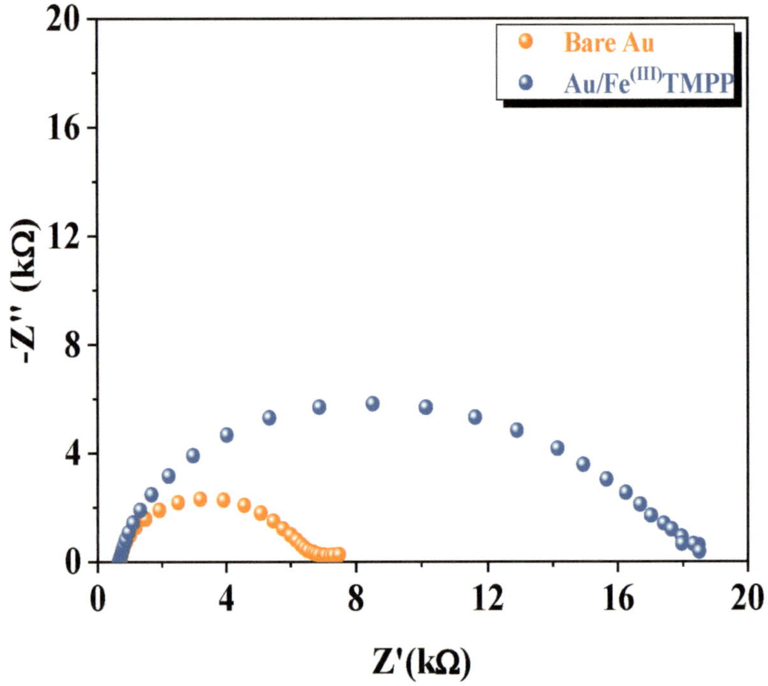

Figure 3.
Nyquist plots of bare Au and Au/Fe$^{(III)}$TMPP in PBS (0.1 M PBS, pH = 7).

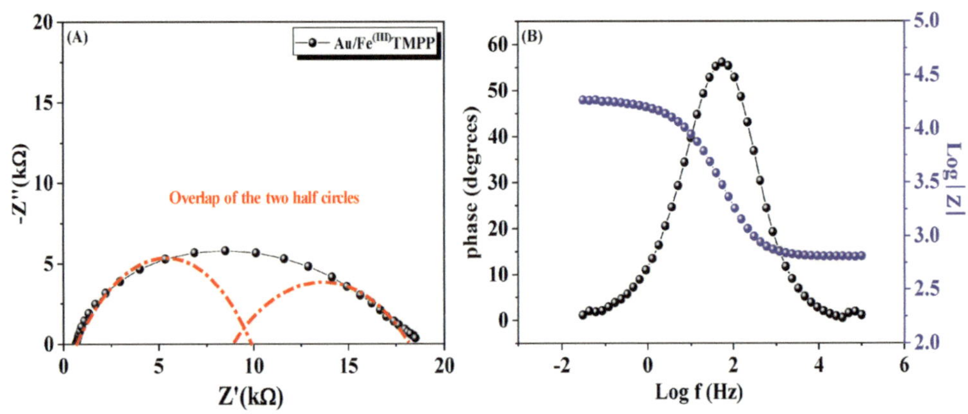

Figure 4.
(A) Nyquist and (B) Bode plots of the Au/Fe$^{(III)}$TMPP electrode with the fit result.

overlap of two closely interacting semicircles [35] which can indicate the presence of more than one dipole in the equivalent electrical circuit model [36]. **Figure 4B** shows the bode diagram fit of Au/Fe$^{(III)}$TMPP electrode. This figure reveals that phase plot presents one phase pic maxima. Consequently, the equivalent electric circuit is analyzed as one dipole [36]. Taking into account the interpretation of Nyquist and bode diagrams of Au/Fe$^{(III)}$TMPP, the best circuit that has been chosen is shown in **Figure 5**. This circuit has shown the best fit with low total error χ^2. This circuit consists of an electrolyte resistance denoted R_s placed in series with one electrical dipole which divides itself into two dipoles. The first dipole is formed by (R_m, CPE1) corresponding to the first high frequency loop and describes the

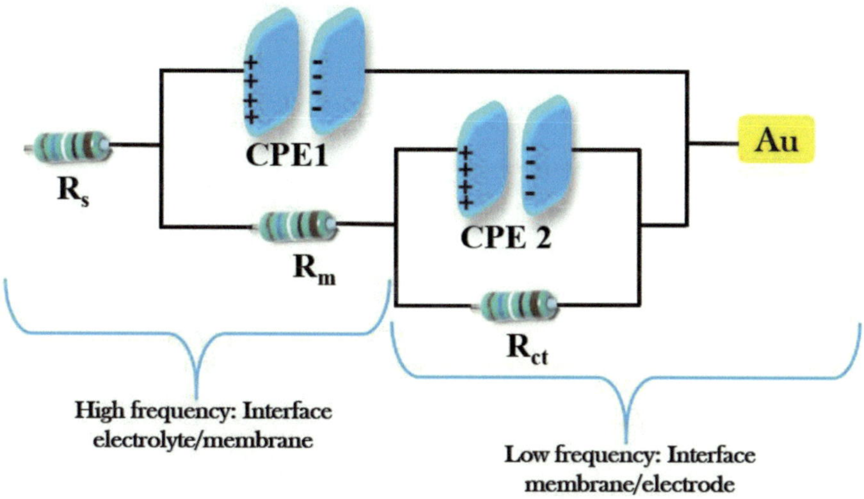

Figure 5.
Equivalent circuit used to fit the impedance spectra of Au/Fe$^{(III)}$TMPP electrode.

electrochemical phenomena occurring at the electrolyte/membrane interface where R_m is the resistance of the membrane and CPE1 is called the constant phase element. The second dipole is made up by (R_{ct}, CPE2) describing the second loop at low frequencies and describes the electrochemical phenomena occurring at the membrane/electrode interface where R_{ct} represents the charge transfer resistance at the membrane/electrode interface.

In our previous optical study, Fe$^{(III)}$TMPP was able to detect BPA molecules through the strong coordination ability of Fe$^{(III)}$ cation to oxygen atoms [26]. Thus, in this study, the Au/Fe$^{(III)}$TMPP electrode has been used to test its ability towards the impedimetric detection of BPA and 2 other interferent molecules. These interfering molecules are 2,2-'biphenol and catechol, which have a structure similar to BPA. The choice of EIS technique to detect these phenolic compounds was made because of its several advantages, such as simplicity, label-free, high sensitivity, and serving as a way to interface recognition events and signal transduction.

BPA is an electron-rich system favorable for the strong interaction with porphyrin ring. Hence, we explore the use of the electrostatic interaction between BPA and cell porphyrin membrane without using any external redox indicator. Thus the detection is directly proportional to the change in the electrical properties of the electroactive Fe$^{(III)}$TMPP membrane. **Figure 6** shows the Nyquist plot of Au/Fe$^{(III)}$TMPP for different BPA, 2,2-'biphenol and catechol concentrations (from 10^{-12} to 10^{-7} M). Au/Fe$^{(III)}$TMPP electrode shows a large increase in diameter of the semicircle, after BPA, 2,2'-biphenol and catechol attachment, correlated with their increasing concentrations, indicating much higher R_{ct} values. This increase can be associated with the multilayer adsorption of BPA, 2,2′-biphenol and catechol molecules on the surface of Fe$^{(III)}$TMPP membrane, which leads to the modification of electrochemical properties at the interface.

To confirm this mechanism of detection, the electrochemical proprieties of the sensor have been quantified by fitting the Nyquist plots using the equivalent circuit shown in **Figure 5**. The different fits are done with a total error value (χ^2) less than 10^{-3}. **Figure 7** shows the variation of the membrane resistance R_m as a function of the BPA, 2,2′-biphenol and catechol concentrations cologarithm $p[X] = -\log[CX]$, where X = BPA, 2,2′-biphenol and catechol. We can observe that the value of R_m increases when increasing the concentration of the three studied analytes.

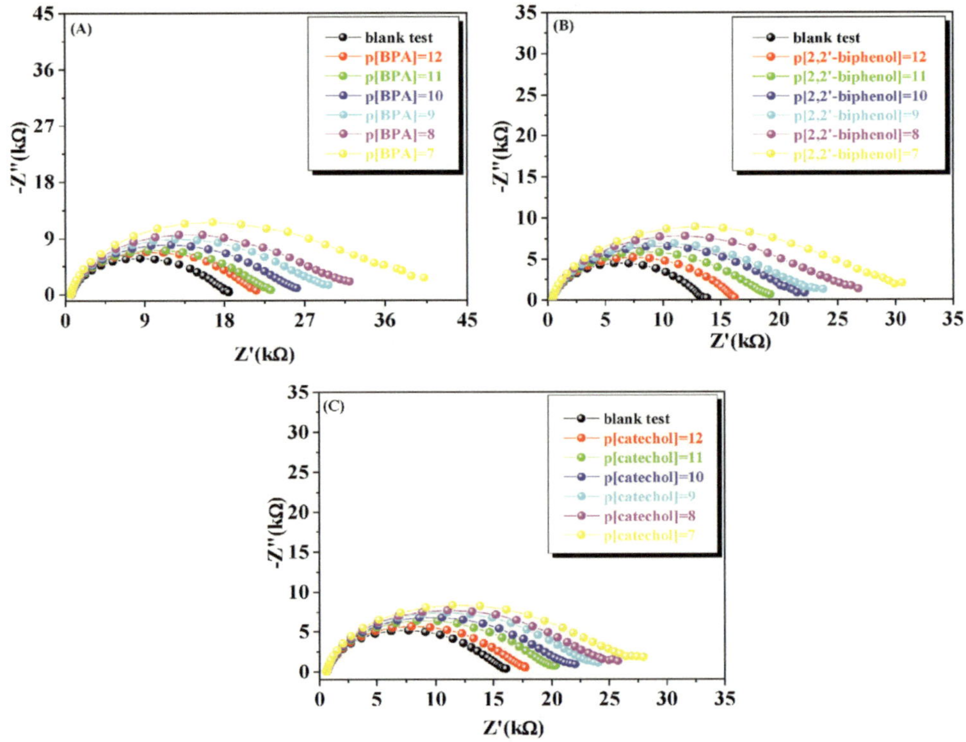

Figure 6.
Nyquist diagrams of Au/Fe$^{(III)}$TMPP electrode for different (A) BPA, (B) 2,2′-biphenol and (C) catechol concentrations in PBS (0.1 M, pH = 7). Frequency range [100 kHz–30mHz]. Potential polarization E = −900 mV. The points presenting the experimental data and the line is the fit obtained with the equivalent circuit shown below.

This result indicates an increase in the thickness of the Fe$^{(III)}$TMPP membrane, which is proportional to R_m according to the following Eq. (1).

$$R_m = \frac{d}{\delta S} \tag{1}$$

Where d is the membrane thickness, δ is the conductivity of the membrane and S the active area.

Consequently, the increase of the thickness of the Fe$^{(III)}$TMPP membrane correlated with the increase of BPA, 2,2′-biphenol and catechol concentrations proves the adsorption of these molecules on the surface of the Fe$^{(III)}$TMPP membrane through their π electron system [37].

To fully understand the charge transfer kinetics at the interfaces, the R_{ct} values after BPA, 2,2′-biphenol and catechol attachment were obtained from the equivalent circuit model and used to generate **Figure 8**. This figure describes the evolution of the charge transfer resistance R_{ct} characteristic of the Au/Fe$^{(III)}$TMPP interface, as a function of the logarithm of the concentration of BPA, 2,2′-biphenol and catechol. We report, from the curve of R_{ct} = f (p [X]), that the charge transfer resistance increased with the increase of BPA, 2,2′-biphenol and catechol concentrations leading to down the electron transfer to Au/Fe$^{(III)}$TMPP electrode. This is due to the steric hindrance favored by the multi layers adsorption of the target molecules, which seems logical since it has been shown from Eq. (1) that the sensitive membrane thickness has already increased upon the increasing of the analyte concentrations.

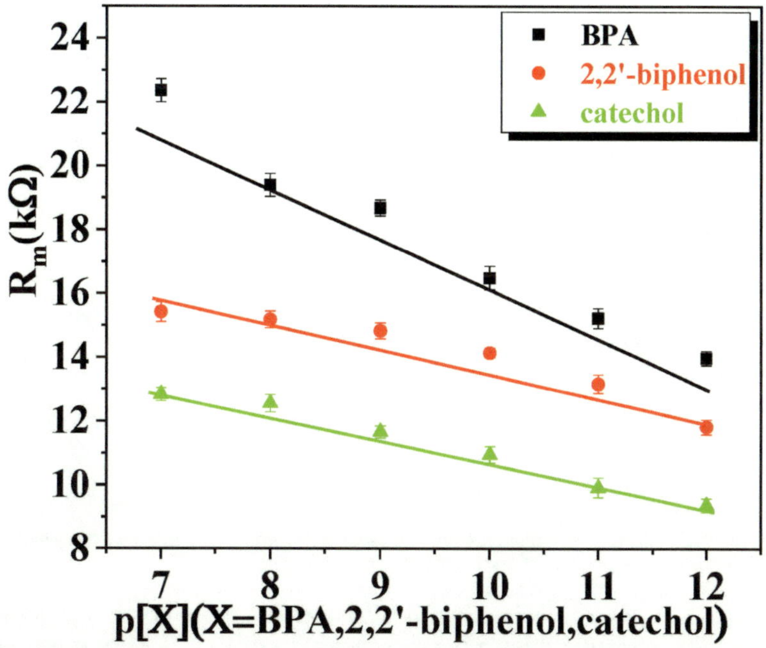

Figure 7.
Variation of the $Fe^{(III)}$TMPP membrane resistance (R_m) plots versus p[X].

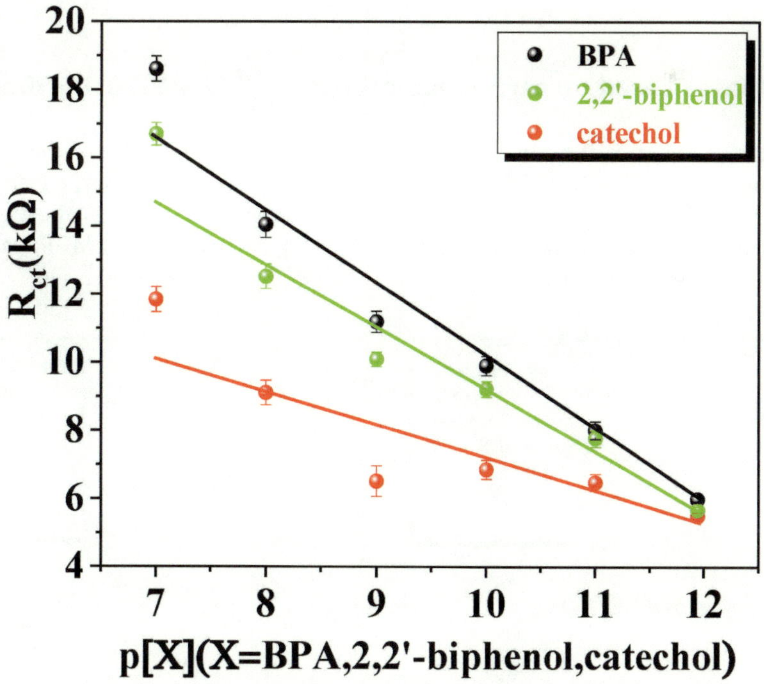

Figure 8.
Variation of the $Fe^{(III)}$TMPP charge transfer resistance (R_{ct}) plots versus p[X].

The R_{ct} slope values of the Au transducer coated by $Fe^{(III)}$TMPP membrane for the impedimetric detection of BPA, 2,2′-biphenol and catechol are illustrated in **Table 1**. As can be seen, the slope associated with the catechol molecule has a lower

Sensitive membrane	Analytes	R_{ct} slope (kΩ/decade)
$Fe^{(III)}$TMPP	bisphenol A	2.104
	2,2′-biphenol	1.770
	catechol	0.983

Table 1.
Comparison of the R_{ct} slope values of Au/$Fe^{(III)}$TMPP electrode for different phenolic analytes.

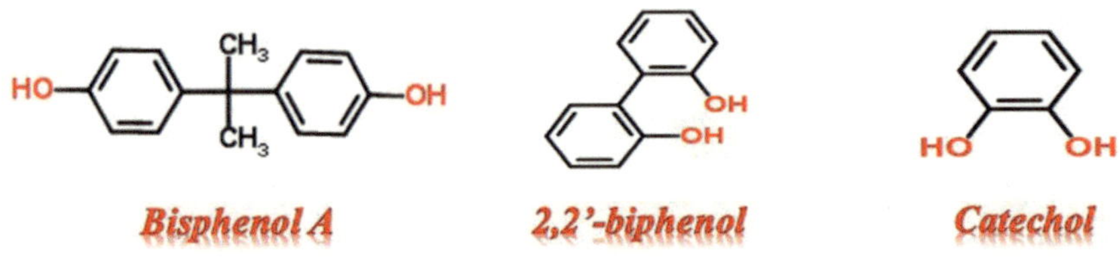

Figure 9.
Chemical structure of BPA, 2,2′-biphenol and catechol showing the presence of two aromatic rings in bisphenol A and 2,2′-biphenol and the presence of one aromatic ring in catechol.

value, whereas the slope associated with BPA and 2,2′-biphenol molecules has a higher value. These results show a better sensitivity of $Fe^{(III)}$TMPP towards BPA molecules. This can be explained by the higher number of aromatic groups in the structures of BPA and 2,2′-biphenol than in the structure of catechol (**Figure 9**). According to these results, we have chosen BPA as the target molecule for $Fe^{(III)}$TMPP membrane throughout our next measurements.

4. BPA sensor based on carbon nanotubes/$Fe^{(III)}$TMPP nanocomposite

In order to enhance the sensitivity of the $Fe^{(III)}$TMPP towards the detection of BPA, carbon nanotubes (CNTs) has been used to dope iron (III) porphyrin as it has attracted considerable interest due to its excellent electrochemical properties and its high ability to amplify the detection signal [38, 39]. Hence, $Fe^{(III)}$TMPP was doped

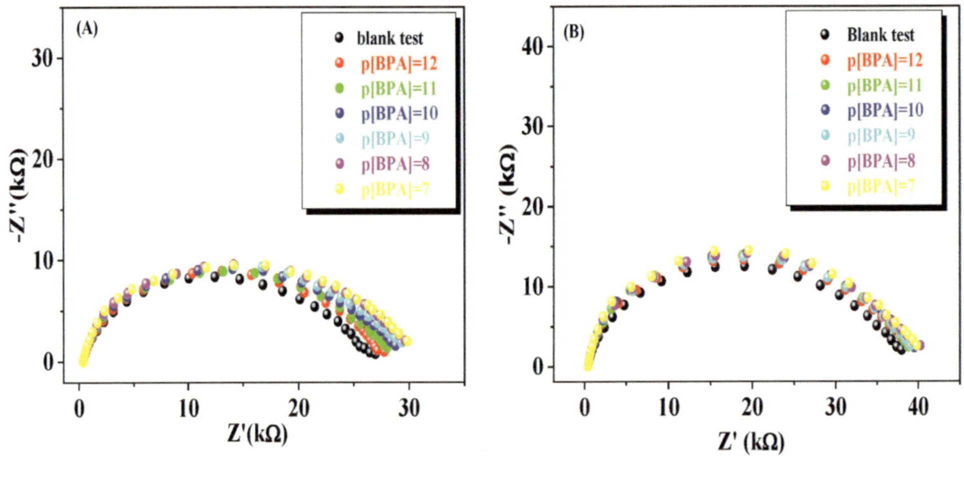

Figure 10.
Nyquist diagrams of (A) Au/2%CNTs/$Fe^{(III)}$TMPP electrode and (B) Au/4%CNTs/$Fe^{(III)}$TMPP electrode for different BPA concentrations.

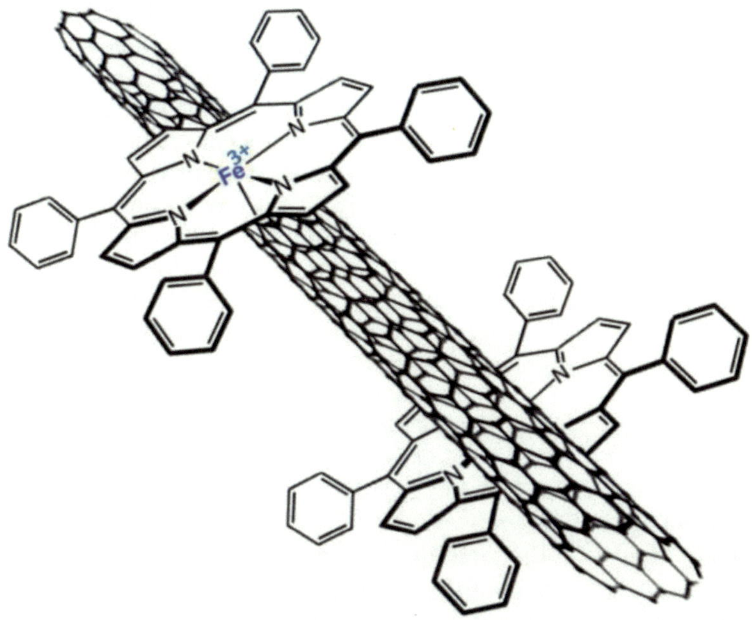

Figure 11.
Schematic presentation of the non-interaction of most aromatic rings of Fe$^{(III)}$TMPP with CNT because of their unsuitable structures.

by 2% CNTs and 4% CNTs, then the obtained 2% CNTs/Fe$^{(III)}$TMPP and 4%CNTs/Fe$^{(III)}$TMPP nanocomposites have been used for the detection of different concentrations of BPA (**Figure 10**). As can be seen, the Nyquist plots of 2%CNTs/Fe$^{(III)}$TMPP and 4%CNTs/Fe$^{(III)}$TMPP modified Au electrodes show a very small variation with increasing BPA concentrations. This result shows that the doping of porphyrin by CNTs did not improve its sensitivity towards the detection of BPA molecules. This can be explained by the planar structure of Fe$^{(III)}$TMPP making difficult the π- π interaction with the rolled up tubular structure of CNT (**Figure 11**). These results led us to think about improving the sensitivity of the Au/Fe$^{(III)}$TMPP sensor using another carbon material having a 2D planar structure which can make easier the π- π interaction with Fe$^{(III)}$TMPP and preserves its structure. Because of its fascinating electronic properties and extremely high specific surface area, this chosen carbon material is known as reduced graphene oxide (RGO), a graphene derivate that has attracted a lot of attention in improving the sensing ability of BPA sensors [40].

5. BPA sensor based on nanocarbon transducer functionalized by Fe$^{(III)}$TMPP

After proving the good affinity of Fe$^{(III)}$TMPP towards BPA molecules, we aim to improve the sensitivity of Au/Fe$^{(III)}$TMPP sensor by involving the use of nanosized electrodes based on nanocarbon transducers. Hence, owing to its strong electrocatalytic activity and minimal surface fouling, RGO has been chosen as a nanocarbon material to functionalize it on Au electrode to form a new Au/RGO nanocarbon transducer with enhanced charge transfer ability than the Au transducer. Then, the Au/RGO nanocarbon transducer has been prepared and functionalized with Fe$^{(III)}$TMPP membrane to form Au/RGO/Fe$^{(III)}$TMPP platform.

With the objective of highlighting the interaction between the $Fe^{(III)}$TMPP and the Au/RGO nanocarbon transducer, UV/vis has been used. Hence, the prepared ITO/RGO, ITO/$Fe^{(III)}$TMPP and ITO/RGO/$Fe^{(III)}$TMPP electrodes were characterized by UV–vis (**Figure 12**). As shown in **Figure 12**, the UV/vis absorption spectrum of ITO/$Fe^{(III)}$TMPP exhibits a strong peak at 438 nm and a weak peak at 527 nm ascribed to the Soret band and the Q-band of porphyrin respectively. After we have deposited the $Fe^{(III)}$TMPP on ITO/RGO, we have observed a decrease in the Soret and Q band intensities with a red shift from 438 nm to 431 nm for the Soret band and the Q-band shift from 527 nm to 536 nm. These shifts prove the strong π-π interactions between the aromatic rings of RGO and the $Fe^{(III)}$TMPP macrocycles [41, 42]. These results confirm the formation of the graphene–porphyrin complex, being in agreement with the proposed hypothesis of the easier interaction of the flattened structure of porphyrin with the 2D surface of graphene (**Figure 13**).

Bare Au, Au/$Fe^{(III)}$TMPP, Au/RGO and Au/RGO/$Fe^{(III)}$TMPP electrodes have been characterized by EIS in PBS (0.1 M, pH = 7) with an optimized potential of −0.9 V (**Figure 14**).

As shown in **Figure 14**, the total impedance plot of Au/RGO shows a semi cercle with a diameter smaller than obtained with bare Au. Consequently, the R_{ct} value of Au/RGO decreased compared to that of bare Au. This result proves that the fabricated Au/RGO nanocarbon transducer has improved charge transfer ability than the usual transducer (Bare Au) thanks to the electron catalyst role of RGO. As illustrated in **Figure 14**, the impedance plot of Au/RGO/$Fe^{(III)}$TMPP structure presents a very smaller semi cercle diameter compared to Au/$Fe^{(III)}$TMPP electrode which is explained by smaller R_{ct} value for Au/RGO/$Fe^{(III)}$TMPP, thus better charge transfer ability at the interface electrode/electrolyte. This result demonstrates that the Au/RGO nanocarbon transducer ensured the good attachment of the porphyrin on its surface via π-π interaction as we have proved by UV–visible which leads to enhanced kinetic charge transfer of the Au/RGO/$Fe^{(III)}$TMPP structure.

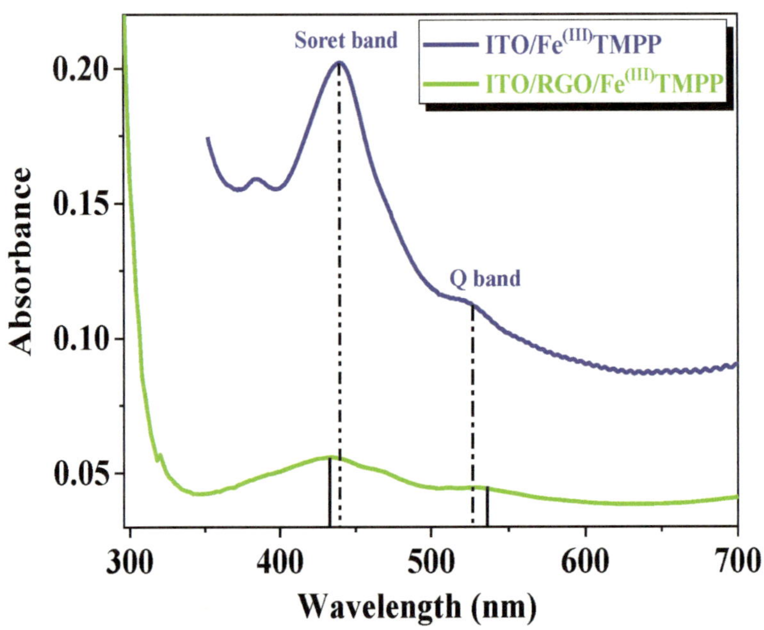

Figure 12.
UV/vis spectra of ITO/$Fe^{(III)}$TMPP and ITO/RGO/$Fe^{(III)}$TMPP structures.

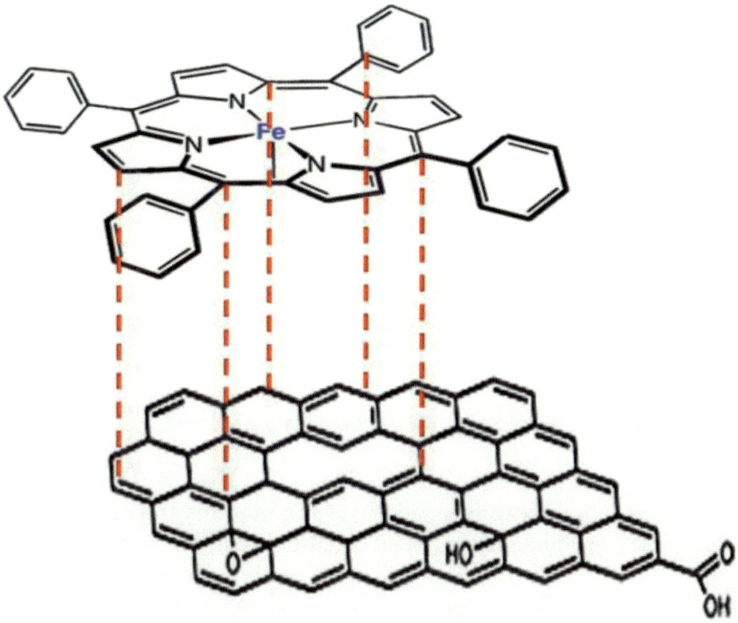

Figure 13.
Schematic presentation of the π-π interaction between aromatic rings of $Fe^{(III)}$*TMPP and RGO thanks to their planar structures.*

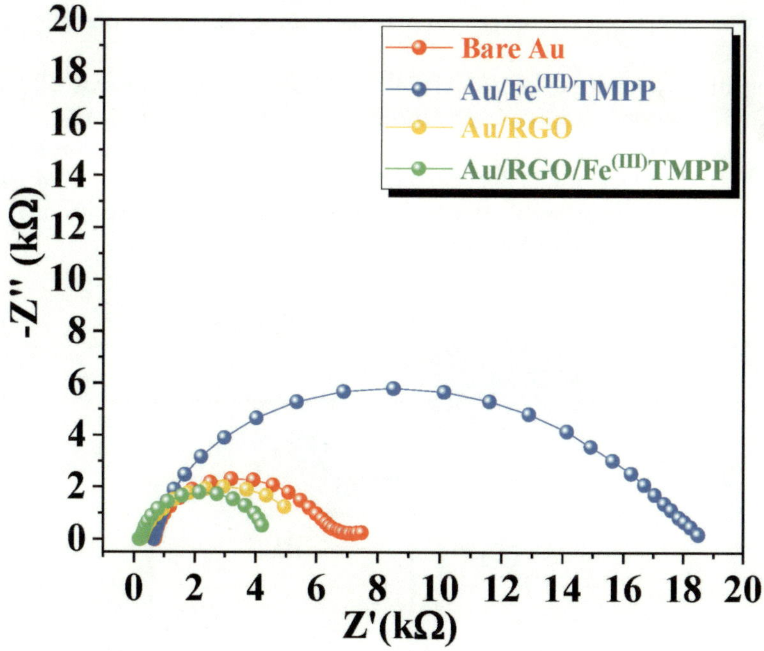

Figure 14.
Nyquist plot of Bare Au, Au/$Fe^{(III)}$*TMPP, Au/RGO and Au/RGO/*$Fe^{(III)}$*TMPP electrodes in PBS (0.1 M, pH = 7).*

The Nyquist diagram of Au/RGO/$Fe^{(III)}$TMPP electrode, as shown in **Figure 15**, reveals the presence of a small semicircle at high frequency, corresponding to a small phase pic maxima in the phase diagram, and a large second semicircle at low

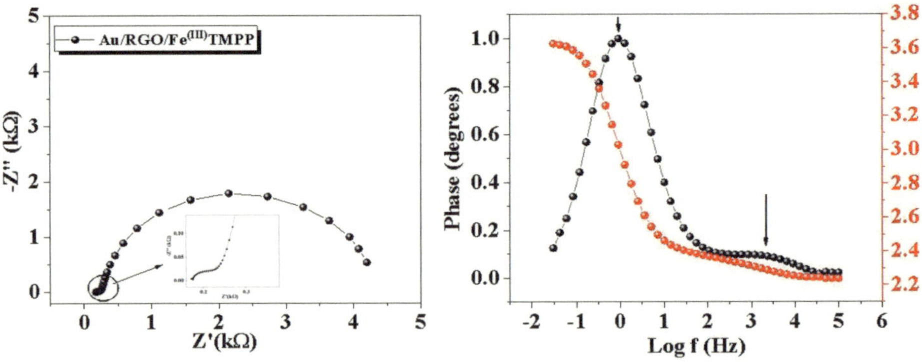

Figure 15.
Nyquist and Bode plots of the Au/RGO/Fe$^{(III)}$TMPP electrode with the fit result.

frequency, corresponding to an intense phase pic maxima in the phase diagram. Hence, the proposed equivalent electrical circuit should be composed by more than one dipole [28]. The best fit was done using an equivalent electrical circuit formed by a parallel association of two dipoles placed in series with the electrolyte resistance (R_s) (**Figure 16**). The first dipole, which is attributed to the high frequency loop and the electrochemical phenomena occurring at the electrolyte/membrane interface, was formed by a membrane resistance (R_m) and a membrane capacitance (C_m). The second dipole, is attributed to the second loop at low frequencies and describes the electrochemical phenomena taking place at the membrane/electrode interface, was composed of charge transfer resistance (R_{ct}) and constant phase element (CPE).

The sensing properties of Au/RGO/Fe$^{(III)}$TMPP electrode towards BPA concentrations in PBS electrolyte have been studied and presented in **Figure 17**. The semicircle diameter related to the charge transfer resistance (R_{ct}) from the RGO/Fe$^{(III)}$TMPP to the electrode is observed to increase upon the addition of BPA concentration. This considerable dependance affirms the high affinity of Au/RGO/Fe$^{(III)}$TMPP sensor towards BPA molecules.

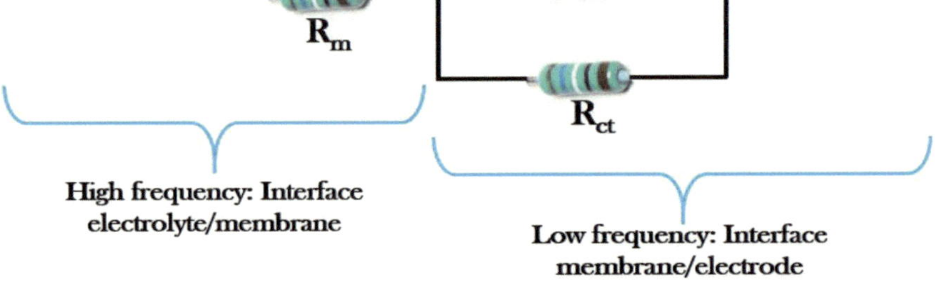

Figure 16.
Equivalent circuit used to fit the impedance spectra of Au/RGO/Fe$^{(III)}$TMPP electrode.

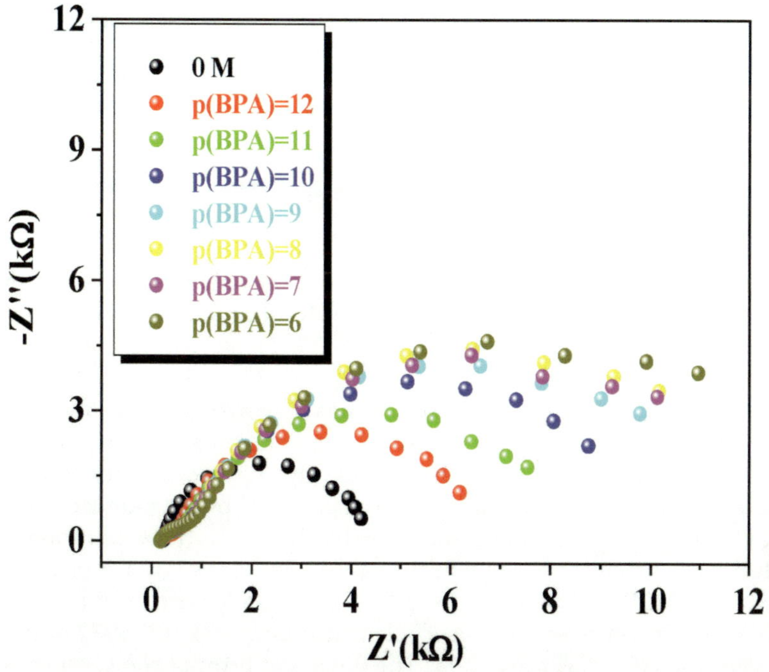

Figure 17.
EIS responses of the Au/RGO/Fe$^{(III)}$TMPP electrode in the absence and the presence of different BPA concentrations.

The electrical parameters values of Au/RGO/Fe$^{(III)}$TMPP electrode after BPA attachment were obtained from the equivalent circuit model presented in **Figure 16.** Then a comparative study of R_m and R_{ct} variations versus p[BPA] for Au/Fe$^{(III)}$TMPP and Au/RGO/Fe$^{(III)}$TMPP electrodes has been studied (**Figure 18**).

As can be observed in **Figure 18**, R_m and R_{ct} variations increase with the successive addition of BPA concentration for the Au/Fe$^{(III)}$TMPP and Au/RGO/Fe$^{(III)}$TMPP electrodes. This result confirms the adsorption mechanism of BPA on the surface of the two modified electrodes, resulting in an increase of their

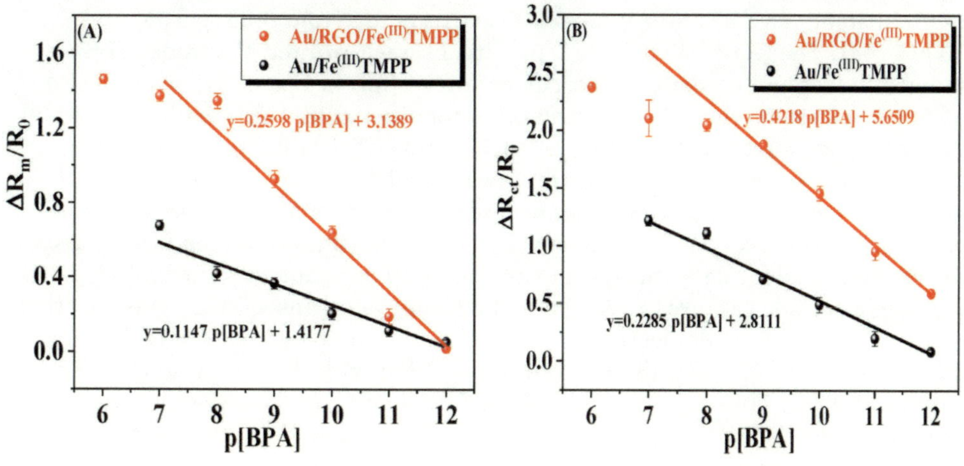

Figure 18.
Variation of the relative changes of (A) the membrane resistance and (B) the charge transfer resistance of Au/Fe$^{(III)}$TMPP and Au/RGO/Fe$^{(III)}$TMPP electrodes versus BPA concentration cologarithm (p[BPA]). $\Delta R_{ct} = R_{ct} - R_{cto}$ where R_{ct} is the charge transfer resistance of the sensing membrane for each BPA concentration and R_{cto} is the charge transfer resistance without any addition of concentration.

Electrodes	Slope of R_m variation	Slope of R_{ct} variation
Au/$Fe^{(III)}$TMPP	0.1147	0.2285
Au/RGO/$Fe^{(III)}$TMPP	0.2598	0.4218

Table 2.
Comparison of the R_m and R_{ct} variations slopes values of Au/$Fe^{(III)}$TMPP and Au/RGO/$Fe^{(III)}$TMPP electrodes for BPA detection.

thickness membranes correlated with a decrease of the electron transfer ability at the membrane/electrode interface. The slope of R_m and R_{ct} variations curves versus p[BPA] for Au/$Fe^{(III)}$TMPP and Au/RGO/$Fe^{(III)}$TMPP electrodes are summarized in **Table 2**. This table shows that the slopes of R_m and R_{ct} variations curves obtained with Au/RGO/$Fe^{(III)}$TMPP electrode are 2 times higher than those obtained with Au/$Fe^{(III)}$TMPP electrode. This result proves the doubled sensitivity with the Au/RGO/$Fe^{(III)}$TMPP electrode towards BPA. This improved sensitivity comes from the catalyst role of RGO [43] which has created a nanocarbon transducer with enhanced electrical property and signal transfer. Based on the calibration curve (**Figure 18B**), the sensitivity (slope of the calibration curve) of our proposed sensor Au/RGO/$Fe^{(III)}$TMPP was found to be 0.4218 per decade with an intercept of 5.6509. The correlation regression coefficient was obtained at 0.9987 in the concentration range from 10^{-12} M to 10^{-8} M. The detection limit of the sensor was estimated to be 2.1 10^{-13} M (signal-to-noise ratio of 3 independent measurements).

6. Comparative study

Because of the biologically harmful and toxicologically relevant of BPA even at low doses, researchers are competing to develop a new electrochemical sensor to track low BPA levels. **Table 3** illustrates a comparison of the analytical performances between our BPA sensor based on RGO nanocarbon transducer (Au/RGO/$Fe^{(III)}$TMPP) and other recently reported BPA sensors. Alam et al. reported graphene oxide and β-cyclodextrin functionalized multiwalled carbon nanotubes (GO-MWCNT-βCD) for the detection of BPA at nanomolar level (6 nM) with good reproducibility (n = 3) and a two-step linear response from 0.05 to 5 μM and 5–30 μM [44]. The GO-MWCNT-βCD modified screen-printed electrode (SPE) showed the highest oxidation peak current of 49.4 μA at Epa of 595 mV for BPA, which is at least 1.6 times higher than other modified SPEs. This was explained by the synergistic effect between GO, MWCNT and βCD leading to a fast electron transfer kinetics, consequently an amplified signal detection of BPA. Wan et al. reported an eco-friendly electrochemical sensor based on Multi-Walled Carbon Nanotubes (MWCNT)/Polythiophene(PTh)/Pt nanocomposites-modified glassy carbon electrode for determination of BPA molecules in aqueous media [45]. The working electrode captures BPA electrochemically and consequently gets adsorbed on the MWCNT-PTh-Pt electrode surface electrode followed by electrochemical oxidation by differential pulse voltammetry (DPV) with the increased oxidation current at 0.5 V. This affinity was explained by the Pt nanocluster that acted as a suitable catalyst of MWCNT-PTh nanocomposite and enhanced the electrochemical detection signal of BPA. Moreover, this sensor platform revealed linear response for BPA detection from 0.005 to 0.4 μM in phosphate buffer saline (PBS) solution and the detection limit was found to be 0.003 μM (S/N = 3). Ponnaiah et al. designed a GCE modified with a new nanocomposite composed of ruthenium nanoparticles, polyaniline and graphitic carbon nitride (Ru^0/PANI/g-C_3N_4) as an electrochemical

Sensor material	Detection method	LOD (μM)	Linear range (μM)	Preparation method of the sensor	Reference
GO-MWCNT-βCD/SPE	LSV	6	0.05–5/5–30	Covalent modification of MWCNTs with βCD/ drop casting of GO-MWCNT-βCD suspension on SPE	[44]
MWCNT/PTh/Pt/GCE	DPV	3.0×10^{-3}	0.005–0.4	Electrodeposition of MWCNT-PTh-Pt on GCE	[45]
Ru^0/PANI@g-C_3N_4	DPV	0.18×10^{-3}	0.01–1.1	Long time ultrasonication of the Ru^0/PANI/g-C_3N_4 nanocomposite / drop casting of Ru^0/PANI/g-C_3N_4 suspension on GCE	[46]
ND-GCE	SWV	13×10^{-3}	0.1–80	Ultrasonication of ND in water followed by drop casting on GCE	[47]
AgNPs-EG	SWV	0.23	5.0–100	Long term preparation of AgNPs-EG electrode	[48]
Au/RGO/$Fe^{(III)}$TMPP	EIS	2.1×10^{-7}	10^{-6}–10^{-2}	Simple and fast ultrasonication of RGO and $Fe^{(III)}$TMPP/drop casting deposition of RGO and $Fe^{(III)}$TMPP on Au electrode respectively	This work

Table 3.
Comparison of the detection method, detection limit, linear range and preparation method of the sensor of recently reported sensors and the present study for the determination of BPA.

sensor for the detection of BPA [46]. The sensor system exhibits picomolar-level detection limits, good sensitivity and stability with a detection range from 0.01 to 1.1 μM. This result was explained by the synergistic effect of the nanocomposite: the high activity of ruthenium nanoparticles, the porous structure of the conducting PANI and the catalyst role of g-C_3N_4 that created an amplified detection system. Jiang et al. reported the development of electrochemical sensors based on carbon nanomaterials, i.e. nanodiamond (ND/GCE) and nanocarbon (NC/GCE) [47]. These carbon materials have achieved a good sensitivity towards BPA monitored by Square Wave Voltammetry (SWV) thanks to their low fouling properties and porous structures. The limit of detection of the proposed sensor was at the nanomolar level with an acceptable liner range from 0.1 to 80 μM. Tsekeli et al. reported the synthesis of silver nanoparticle-exfoliated graphite nanocomposite (AgNPs-EG) for the application of BPA sensor [48]. The AgNPs-EG nanocomposite-based electrode has demonstrated antifouling property and acceptable affinity towards BPA with LOD of 0.23 μM and a linear range from 5.0 to 100 μM.

Compared with all these recently reported BPA sensors (**Table 3**), our work based on Au/RGO/$Fe^{(III)}$TMPP sensor presents the best sensing platform because of its lower limit of detection in the picomolar level (2.1 10^{-7} μM) and wider linear range spreading from 10^{-6} to 10^{-2} μM. Hence, the sensor based on nanocarbon transducer functionalized by $Fe^{(III)}$TMPP presented in this work is capable of measuring BPA at concentrations lower than the daily dose limits set by recent medical advice. In addition to a lower detection limit and wide detection range, our fabrication method is based only on drop-casting and drying, which is more facile and less time consuming than other methods. Furthermore, the modification of our sensor is based on non-covalent bonding which preserves the sp^2 structures of each membrane, leading to a good stability of the BPA response signal. Another advantage of our proposed sensor was that, in our work, electrochemical impedance spectroscopy was used to follow the detection signal of BPA, while it was rarely used compared to DPV and SWV methods to monitor the attachment of BPA on the sensor surface. The advantage of the EIS method compared to the most frequently used SWV and DPV methods is that it does not damage the electrode surface and also enables low detection limits [49].We envisage that such sensors are promising tools to face the challenges of the detection of BPA at trace level in aqueous media, as an alternative to the conventional test or central lab equipment.

The better sensing performance of our sensor based on Au/RGO/$Fe^{(III)}$TMPP could be attributed to different aspects such as the architecture of the modified electrode that is based on Au/RGO nanocarbon transducer for immobilized $Fe^{(III)}$TMPP to retain its stability and activity which can facilitate the reaction towards BPA. Moreover, the high electric conductivity of RGO nanocarbon material can create a novel nanocarbon transducer with higher kinetic charge transfer compared to usual used transducers which facilitates the mediation of electrocommunication between the BPA and the electrode.

7. Conclusions

In this chapter, a label-free impedimetric sensor using Au/RGO nanocarbon transducer functionalized by $Fe^{(III)}$TMPP has been successfully designed for the detection of trace BPA. The Au/RGO/$Fe^{(III)}$TMPP electrode was fabricated by loading RGO and $Fe^{(III)}$TMPP membrane on Au transducer, respectively. The Au/RGO/$Fe^{(III)}$TMPP sensor has demonstrated an amplified response towards BPA compared to that of Au/$Fe^{(III)}$TMPP electrode. This enhancement was attributed to the Au/RGO nanocarbon transducer which acted as a charge transfer catalyst and good platform for the attachment of $Fe^{(III)}$TMPP via π- π staking. The suggested Au/RGO/$Fe^{(III)}$TMPP has offered a few advantages compared to the previously reported strategy for the determination of BPA, including excellent low LOD (2.1 10^{-13} M) and wide linear dynamic range with a simple and efficient fabrication method. The findings from this study will be valuable for constructing highly sensitive sensors based on modified Au/RGO nanocarbon transducer to detect various substances with low concentration and trace amount.

Author details

Zouhour Hsine* and Rym Mlika
Laboratory of Interfaces and Advanced Materials, Faculty of Science of Monastir, University of Monastir, Monastir, Tunisia

*Address all correspondence to: zouhourhsine1@gmail.com

References

[1] Lee E-H, Lim HJ, Lee S-D, Son A. Highly Sensitive Detection of Bisphenol A by NanoAptamer Assay with Truncated Aptamer. ACS Appl Mater Interfaces 2017;9:14889–98. https://doi.org/10.1021/acsami.7b02377.

[2] Liu Y, Yao L, He L, Liu N, Piao Y. Electrochemical Enzyme Biosensor Bearing Biochar Nanoparticle as Signal Enhancer for Bisphenol A Detection in Water. Sensors (Basel) 2019;19. https://doi.org/10.3390/s19071619.

[3] Kazane I, Gorgy K, Gondran C, Spinelli N, Zazoua A, Defrancq E, et al. Highly Sensitive Bisphenol-A Electrochemical Aptasensor Based on Poly(Pyrrole-Nitrilotriacetic Acid)-Aptamer Film. Anal Chem 2016;88: 7268–73. https://doi.org/10.1021/acs.analchem.6b01574.

[4] Manna B. Rational functionalization of reduced graphene oxide with an imidazole group for the electrochemical sensing of bisphenol A - an endocrine disruptor. Analyst 2018;143:3451–7. https://doi.org/10.1039/c8an00642c.

[5] Zainul R, Abd Azis N, Md Isa I, Hashim N, Ahmad MS, Saidin MI, et al. Zinc/Aluminium–Quinclorac Layered Nanocomposite Modified Multi-Walled Carbon Nanotube Paste Electrode for Electrochemical Determination of Bisphenol A. Sensors 2019;19:941. https://doi.org/10.3390/s19040941.

[6] Li X, Huang Y, Chen M, Tong Y, Zhang C. A label-free electrochemical bisphenol A immunosensor based on chlorogenic acid as a redox probe. Anal Methods 2017;9:2183–8. https://doi.org/10.1039/C6AY02997C.

[7] Song Y, Xu M, Li Z, He L, Hu M, He L, et al. Ultrasensitive detection of bisphenol A under diverse environments with an electrochemical aptasensor based on multicomponent AgMo heteronanostructure. Sensors and Actuators B: Chemical 2020;321:128527. https://doi.org/10.1016/j.snb.2020.128527.

[8] Kesavan G, Nataraj N, Chen S-M, Lin L-H. Hydrothermal synthesis of NiFe2O4 nanoparticles as an efficient electrocatalyst for the electrochemical detection of bisphenol A. New J Chem 2020;44:7698–707. https://doi.org/10.1039/D0NJ00608D.

[9] Wang X, Li Y, Zhou Y, He Y. Application of a novel endocrine disruptor bisphenol A electrochemical sensor based on analogous heterostructure characteristics of La-doped Yb2O3 nanomaterials. Anal Methods 2019;11:5613–22. https://doi.org/10.1039/C9AY01694E.

[10] Ali H, Mukhopadhyay S, Jana NR. Selective electrochemical detection of bisphenol A using a molecularly imprinted polymer nanocomposite. New J Chem 2019;43:1536–43. https://doi.org/10.1039/C8NJ05883K.

[11] Lu YC, Xiao WW, Wang JY, Xiong XH. Rapid isolation and determination of bisphenol A in complicated matrices by magnetic molecularly imprinted electrochemical sensing. Anal Bioanal Chem 2021;413: 389–401. https://doi.org/10.1007/s00216-020-03006-8.

[12] Ben Messaoud N, Ait Lahcen A, Dridi C, Amine A. Ultrasound assisted magnetic imprinted polymer combined sensor based on carbon black and gold nanoparticles for selective and sensitive electrochemical detection of Bisphenol A. Sensors and Actuators B: Chemical 2018;276:304–12. https://doi.org/10.1016/j.snb.2018.08.092.

[13] Yu Z, Luan Y, Li H, Wang W, Wang X, Zhang Q. A disposable electrochemical aptasensor using single-

stranded DNA–methylene blue complex as signal-amplification platform for sensitive sensing of bisphenol A. Sensors and Actuators B: Chemical 2019;284:73–80. https://doi.org/10.1016/j.snb.2018.12.126.

[14] Huang X, Huang D, Chen J, Ye R, Lin Q, Chen S. Fabrication of novel electrochemical sensor based on bimetallic Ce-Ni-MOF for sensitive detection of bisphenol A. Anal Bioanal Chem 2020;412:849–60. https://doi.org/10.1007/s00216-019-02282-3.

[15] Carbone M, Micheli L, Limosani F, Possanza F, Abdallah Y, Tagliatesta P. Ruthenium and manganese metalloporphyrins modified screen-printed electrodes for bio-relevant electroactive targets. J Porphyrins Phthalocyanines 2018;22:491–500. https://doi.org/10.1142/S1088424618500402.

[16] Sakthinathan S, Kubendhiran S, Chen SM, Manibalan K, Govindasamy M, Tamizhdurai P, et al. Reduced Graphene Oxide Non-covalent Functionalized with Zinc Tetra Phenyl Porphyrin Nanocomposite for Electrochemical Detection of Dopamine in Human Serum and Rat Brain Samples. Electroanalysis 2016;28:2126–35. https://doi.org/10.1002/elan.201600085.

[17] Mashazi PN, Nombona N, Muchindu M, Vilakazi S. Metallophthalocyanines and metalloporphyrins as electrocatalysts: a case of hydrogen peroxide and glucose detection. J Porphyrins Phthalocyanines 2012;16:741–53. https://doi.org/10.1142/S1088424612300066.

[18] Jemmeli D, Mchiri C, Dridi C, Nasri H, Dempsey E. Development of a new bisphenol A electrochemical sensor based on a cadmium(II) porphyrin modified carbon paste electrode. RSC Adv 2020;10:31740–7. https://doi.org/10.1039/D0RA04793G.

[19] Negut CC, Staden R-IS- van, Staden JF van. Porphyrins-as Active Materials in the Design of Sensors. An Overview. ECS J Solid State Sci Technol 2020;9:051005. https://doi.org/10.1149/2162-8777/ab9a5d.

[20] Salimi A, MamKhezri H, Hallaj R, Zandi S. Modification of glassy carbon electrode with multi-walled carbon nanotubes and iron(III)-porphyrin film: Application to chlorate, bromate and iodate detection. Electrochimica Acta 2007;52:6097–105. https://doi.org/10.1016/j.electacta.2007.03.046.

[21] Li J, Tu W, Lei J, Tang S, Ju H. Porphyrin-functionalized gold nanoparticles for selective electrochemical detection of peroxyacetic acid. Electrochimica Acta 2011;56:3159–63. https://doi.org/10.1016/j.electacta.2011.01.060.

[22] Wang C, Yuan R, Chai Y, Chen S, Zhang Y, Hu F, et al. Non-covalent iron (III)-porphyrin functionalized multi-walled carbon nanotubes for the simultaneous determination of ascorbic acid, dopamine, uric acid and nitrite. Electrochimica Acta 2012;62:109–15. https://doi.org/10.1016/j.electacta.2011.11.115.

[23] Huang N, Liu M, Li H, Zhang Y, Yao S. Synergetic signal amplification based on electrochemical reduced graphene oxide-ferrocene derivative hybrid and gold nanoparticles as an ultra-sensitive detection platform for bisphenol A. Analytica Chimica Acta 2015;853:249–57. https://doi.org/10.1016/j.aca.2014.10.016.

[24] Kumar DR, Dhakal G, Nguyen VQ, Shim J-J. Molecularly imprinted hornlike polymer@electrochemically reduced graphene oxide electrode for the highly selective determination of an antiemetic drug. Analytica Chimica Acta 2021;1141:71–82. https://doi.org/10.1016/j.aca.2020.10.014.

[25] Bezzon VDN, Montanheiro TLA, de Menezes BRC, Ribas RG, Righetti VAN, Rodrigues KF, et al. Carbon Nanostructure-based Sensors: A Brief Review on Recent Advances. Advances in Materials Science and Engineering 2019;2019:e4293073. https://doi.org/10.1155/2019/4293073.

[26] Zahou I, Hassen LBH, Mlika R, Ben Chaabane R, Nasri H, Ouada HB. Synthesis and investigation on optical and electrical properties of a triflato iron porphyrin: Application as an optical BPA sensor. Synthetic Metals 2016;221: 75–85. https://doi.org/10.1016/j.synthmet.2016.07.020.

[27] Hsine Z, Bizid S, Mlika R, Sauriat-Dorizon H, Haj Said A, Korri-Youssoufi H. Nanocomposite Based on Poly (para-phenylene)/Chemical Reduced Graphene Oxide as a Platform for Simultaneous Detection of Ascorbic Acid, Dopamine and Uric Acid. Sensors 2020;20:1256. https://doi.org/10.3390/s20051256.

[28] Mlika R, Hbaieb S, Ben Chaabene R, Chevalier Y, Kalfat R, Ben Ouada H. Electrochemical properties of gold electrodes functionalized by new pseudo-polyrotaxanes of polyaniline and chemically modified β-cyclodextrin inclusion complex. Synthetic Metals 2012;162:186–92. https://doi.org/10.1016/j.synthmet.2011.11.029.

[29] Touzi H, Chevalier Y, Martin M, Ben Ouada H, Jaffrezic-Renault N. Detection of Gadolinium with an Impedimetric Platform Based on Gold Electrodes Functionalized by 2-Methylpyridine-Substituted Cyclam. Sensors 2021;21:1658. https://doi.org/10.3390/s21051658.

[30] Erdem A, Congur G, Mayer G. Aptasensor platform based on carbon nanofibers enriched screen printed electrodes for impedimetric detection of thrombin. Journal of Electroanalytical Chemistry 2015;758:12–9. https://doi.org/10.1016/j.jelechem.2015.10.002.

[31] Mahmoud A, Echabaane M, Omri K, El Mir L, Ben Chaabane R. Development of an impedimetric non enzymatic sensor based on ZnO and Cu doped ZnO nanoparticles for the detection of glucose. Journal of Alloys and Compounds 2019;786:960–8. https://doi.org/10.1016/j.jallcom.2019.02.060.

[32] da Silva W, Ghica ME, Ajayi RF, Iwuoha EI, Brett CMA. Impedimetric sensor for tyramine based on gold nanoparticle doped-poly(8-anilino-1-naphthalene sulphonic acid) modified gold electrodes. Talanta 2019;195:604–12. https://doi.org/10.1016/j.talanta.2018.11.054.

[33] Bolat G, Vural OA, Yaman YT, Abaci S. Polydopamine nanoparticles-assisted impedimetric sensor towards label-free lung cancer cell detection. Materials Science and Engineering: C 2021;119:111549. https://doi.org/10.1016/j.msec.2020.111549.

[34] Elgiddawy N, Ren S, Ghattas W, Rouby WMAE, El-Gendy AO, Farghali AA, et al. Antimicrobial Activity of Cationic Poly(3-hexylthiophene) Nanoparticles Coupled with Dual Fluorescent and Electrochemical Sensing: Theragnostic Prospect. Sensors 2021;21:1715. https://doi.org/10.3390/s21051715.

[35] Ebdelli R, Rouis A, Mlika R, Bonnamour I, Jaffrezic-Renault N, Ben Ouada H, et al. Electrochemical impedance detection of Hg2+, Ni2+ and Eu3+ ions by a new azo-calix[4]arene membrane. Journal of Electroanalytical Chemistry 2011;661:31–8. https://doi.org/10.1016/j.jelechem.2011.07.007.

[36] Mlika R, Rouis A, Bonnamour I, Ouada HB. Impedance spectroscopic investigation of the effect of thin azo-calix[4]arene film type on the cation sensitivity of the gold electrodes.

Materials Science and Engineering: C 2011;31:1466–71. https://doi.org/10.1016/j.msec.2011.05.017.

[37] Roales J, Pedrosa JM, Guillén MG, Lopes-Costa T, Pinto SMA, Calvete MJF, et al. Optical detection of amine vapors using ZnTriad porphyrin thin films. Sensors and Actuators B: Chemical 2015; 210:28–35. https://doi.org/10.1016/j.snb.2014.12.080.

[38] Ali MY, Alam AU, Howlader MMR. Fabrication of highly sensitive Bisphenol A electrochemical sensor amplified with chemically modified multiwall carbon nanotubes and β-cyclodextrin. Sensors and Actuators B: Chemical 2020;320:128319. https://doi.org/10.1016/j.snb.2020.128319.

[39] Mo F, Xie J, Wu T, Liu M, Zhang Y, Yao S. A sensitive electrochemical sensor for bisphenol A on the basis of the AuPd incorporated carboxylic multi-walled carbon nanotubes. Food Chemistry 2019;292:253–9. https://doi.org/10.1016/j.foodchem.2019.04.034.

[40] Akilarasan M, Kogularasu S, Chen S-M, Chen T-W, Lin S-H. One-step synthesis of reduced graphene oxide sheathed zinc oxide nanoclusters for the trace level detection of bisphenol A in tissue papers. Ecotoxicol Environ Saf 2018;161:699–705. https://doi.org/10.1016/j.ecoenv.2018.06.045.

[41] Chen Y, Mei T, Chen Y, Wang J, Li J, Fu Y, et al. A sensitive porphyrin/reduced graphene oxide electrode for simultaneous detection of guanine and adenine. J Solid State Electrochem 2016; 20:2055–62. https://doi.org/10.1007/s10008-016-3214-7.

[42] Xie H, Li Y-T, Lei Y-M, Liu Y-L, Xiao M-M, Gao C, et al. Real-Time Monitoring of Nitric Oxide at Single-Cell Level with Porphyrin-Functionalized Graphene Field-Effect Transistor Biosensor. Anal Chem 2016; 88:11115–22. https://doi.org/10.1021/acs.analchem.6b03208.

[43] Yang S, Zhang F, Liang Q, Wang Z. A three-dimensional graphene-based ratiometric signal amplification aptasensor for MUC1 detection. Biosensors and Bioelectronics 2018;120: 85–92. https://doi.org/10.1016/j.bios.2018.08.036.

[44] Alam AU, Deen MJ. Bisphenol A Electrochemical Sensor Using Graphene Oxide and β-Cyclodextrin-Functionalized Multi-Walled Carbon Nanotubes. Anal Chem 2020;92:5532–9. https://doi.org/10.1021/acs.analchem.0c00402.

[45] Wan J, Si Y, Li C, Zhang K. Bisphenol a electrochemical sensor based on multi-walled carbon nanotubes/polythiophene/Pt nanocomposites modified electrode. Anal Methods 2016;8:3333–8. https://doi.org/10.1039/C6AY00850J.

[46] Ponnaiah SK, Prakash P, Muthupandian S. Ultrasonic energy-assisted in-situ synthesis of Ru0/PANI/g-C3N4 nanocomposite: Application for picomolar-level electrochemical detection of endocrine disruptor (Bisphenol-A) in humans and animals. Ultrasonics Sonochemistry 2019;58:104629. https://doi.org/10.1016/j.ultsonch.2019.104629.

[47] Jiang L, Santiago I, Foord J. A comparative study of fouling-free nanodiamond and nanocarbon electrochemical sensors for sensitive bisphenol A detection. Carbon 2021;174: 390–5. https://doi.org/10.1016/j.carbon.2020.11.073.

[48] Tsekeli TR, Sebokolodi TI, Karimi-Maleh H, Arotiba OA. A Silver-Loaded Exfoliated Graphite Nanocomposite Anti-Fouling Electrochemical Sensor for Bisphenol A in Thermal Paper Samples. ACS Omega 2021;6:9401–9. https://doi.org/10.1021/acsomega.0c05836.

[49] Yaman YT, Vural OA, Bolat G, Abaci S. One-pot synthesized gold nanoparticle- peptide nanotube modified disposable sensor for impedimetric recognition of miRNA 410. Sensors and Actuators B: Chemical 2020;320:128343. https://doi.org/10.1016/j.snb.2020.128343.